Pharmacogenomics and Precision Medicine

Editors

KRISTEN K. REYNOLDS
ROLAND VALDES Jr

CLINICS IN LABORATORY MEDICINE

www.labmed.theclinics.com

September 2016 • Volume 36 • Number 3

ELSEVIER

1600 John F. Kennedy Boulevard • Suite 1800 • Philadelphia, Pennsylvania, 19103-2899

http://www.theclinics.com

CLINICS IN LABORATORY MEDICINE Volume 36, Number 3
September 2016 ISSN 0272-2712, ISBN-13: 978-0-323-46259-4

Editor: Lauren Boyle
Developmental Editor: Colleen Viola

Reprints. For copies of 100 or more, of articles in this publication, please contact the Commercial Reprints Department, Elsevier Inc., 360 Park Avenue South, New York, New York 10010-1710. Tel. 212-633-3874, Fax: 212-633-3820, E-mail: reprints@elsevier.com.

Clinics in Laboratory Medicine (ISSN 0272-2712) is published quarterly by Elsevier Inc., 360 Park Avenue South, New York, NY 10010-1710. Months of issue are March, June, September, and December. Business and Editorial offices: 1600 John F. Kennedy Blvd., Suite 1800, Philadelphia, PA 19103-2899. Periodicals postage paid at NewYork, NY and additional mailing offices. Subscription prices are $250.00 per year (US individuals), $469.00 per year (US institutions), $100.00 per year (US students), $305.00 per year (Canadian individuals), $570.00 per year (Canadian institutions), $185.00 per year (Canadian students), $390.00 per year (international individuals), $570.00 per year (international institutions), $185.00 (international students). Foreign air speed delivery is included in all Clinics subscription prices. All prices are subject to change without notice. POSTMASTER: Send address changes to *Clinics in Laboratory Medicine*, Elsevier Health Sciences Division, Subscription Customer Service, 3251 Riverport Lane, Maryland Heights, MO 63043. **Customer Service: 1-800-654-2452 (US). From outside of the US and Canada, call 1-314-447-8871. Fax: 1-314-447-8029. E-mail: journalscustomerservice-usa@elsevier.com (for print support) or journalsonlinesupport-usa@elsevier.com (for online support).**

Clinics in Laboratory Medicine is covered in *EMBASE/Exerpta Medica, MEDLINE/PubMed (Index Medicus), Cinahl, Current Contents/Clinical Medicine, BIOSIS* and *ISI/BIOMED*.

Contributors

EDITORS

KRISTEN K. REYNOLDS, PhD
Assistant Clinical Professor, Department of Pathology and Laboratory Medicine, University of Louisville School of Medicine; VP Laboratory Operations, PGXL Laboratories, Louisville, Kentucky

ROLAND VALDES Jr, PhD, DABCC, FACB
Professor of Pathology and Laboratory Medicine and of Biochemistry and Molecular Genetics; Chief, Clinical Chemistry and Toxicology, University of Louisville School of Medicine, Louisville, Kentucky

AUTHORS

INNA BELFER, MD, PhD
Adjunct Associate Professor, Departments of Medicine and Human Genetics, University of Pittsburgh, Pittsburgh, Pennsylvania

JAMES A. BOIANI, MS, JD
Partner, Epstein Becker and Green, PC, Washington, DC

ALEXANDER DUNCAN, MD
Department of Pathology and Laboratory Medicine, Emory University Hospital, Emory University School of Medicine, Atlanta, Georgia

PEGGY L. EL-MALLAKH, PhD
Assistant Professor; Coordinator, Graduate Psychiatric-Mental Health Nursing Program, University of Kentucky College of Nursing, University of Kentucky, Lexington, Kentucky

RIF S. EL-MALLAKH, MD
Professor and Director, Mood Disorders Research Program, Department of Psychiatry and Behavioral Sciences, University of Louisville HealthCare OutPatient Center, University of Louisville School of Medicine, Louisville, Kentucky

LILLIAN JAN FINDLAY, PhD
Assistant Professor, Graduate Psychiatric-Mental Health Nursing Program, University of Kentucky College of Nursing, University of Kentucky, Lexington, Kentucky

CHARLES E. HILL, MD, PhD
Department of Pathology and Laboratory Medicine, Emory University Hospital, Emory University School of Medicine, Atlanta, Georgia

MARK W. LINDER, PhD, DABCC
Executive Vice President, PGXL Laboratories; Professor, Department of Pathology and Laboratory Medicine, University of Louisville School of Medicine, Louisville, Kentucky

CHERYL L. MAIER, MD, PhD
Department of Pathology and Laboratory Medicine, Emory University Hospital, Emory University School of Medicine, Atlanta, Georgia

BETH A. McNALLY, PhD
Senior Scientist, PGXL Laboratories, Louisville, Kentucky

LORI M. MILLNER, PhD, NRCC
Assistant Director of Sequencing Services, PGXL Technologies; Scientist, Department of Pathology and Laboratory Medicine, University of Louisville, Louisville, Kentucky

KRISTEN K. REYNOLDS, PhD
Assistant Clinical Professor, Department of Pathology and Laboratory Medicine, University of Louisville School of Medicine; VP Laboratory Operations, PGXL Laboratories, Louisville, Kentucky

R. JEANNIE ROBERTS, MD
Assistant Professor; Director of Consultation Services, Department of Psychiatry and Behavioral Sciences, University of Louisville HealthCare OutPatient Center, University of Louisville Hospital, University of Louisville School of Medicine, Louisville, Kentucky

GUALBERTO RUAÑO, MD, PhD
Genomas Inc., Hartford, Connecticut

BONNIE I. SCOTT, JD
Associate, Epstein Becker and Green, PC, Washington, DC

RICHARD SEIP, PhD
Sanofi Genzyme, Cambridge, Massachusetts

LINDSAY N. STROTMAN, PhD
Research Scientist, PGXL Technologies; Instructor, Department of Engineering, University of Louisville, Louisville, Kentucky

BRADLEY MERRILL THOMPSON, MBA, JD
Partner, Epstein Becker and Green, PC, Washington, DC

PAUL D. THOMPSON, MD
Division of Cardiology, Hartford Hospital, Hartford, Connecticut

ROLAND VALDES Jr, PhD, DABCC, FACB
Professor of Pathology and Laboratory Medicine and of Biochemistry and Molecular Genetics; Chief, Clinical Chemistry and Toxicology, University of Louisville School of Medicine, Louisville, Kentucky

LYNN R. WEBSTER, MD
Vice President of Scientific Affairs, PRA Health Sciences, Salt Lake City, Utah

FREDERICK WEITENDORF, RN, RPh
Critical Care Clinical Pharmacist, Robley Rex Veterans Affairs Medical Center; Consulting Pharmacist, PGXL Laboratories, Louisville, Kentucky

ANDREAS WINDEMUTH, PhD
Cyclica Inc., Cambridge, Massachusetts

ALAN H.B. WU, PhD
Department of Laboratory Medicine, San Francisco General Hospital, San Francisco, California

DeLU (TYLER) YIN, PhD
Department of Pathology and Laboratory Medicine, University of Louisville School of Medicine, Louisville, Kentucky

Contents

This article introduces fundamental principles of pharmacogenetics as applied to personalized and precision medicine. Pharmacogenetics establishes relationships between pharmacology and genetics by connecting phenotypes and genotypes in predicting the response of therapeutics in individual patients. We describe differences between precision and personalized medicine and relate principles of pharmacokinetics and pharmacodynamics to applications in laboratory medicine. We also review basic principles of pharmacogenetics, including its evolution, how it enables the practice of personalized therapeutics, and the role of the clinical laboratory. These fundamentals are a segue for understanding specific clinical applications of pharmacogenetics described in subsequent articles in this issue.

Certain antithrombotic drugs exhibit high patient-to-patient variability that significantly impacts the safety and efficacy of therapy. Pharmacogenetics offers the possibility of tailoring drug treatment to patients based on individual genotypes, and this type of testing has been recommended for two oral antithrombotic agents, warfarin and clopidogrel, to influence use and guide dosing. Limited studies have identified polymorphisms that affect the metabolism and activity of newer oral antithrombotic drugs, without clear evidence of the clinical relevance of such polymorphisms. This article provides an overview of the current status of pharmacogenetics in oral antithrombotic therapy.

Statin responsiveness is an area of great research interest given the success of the drug class in the treatment of hypercholesterolemia and in primary and secondary prevention of cardiovascular disease. Interrogation of the patient's genome for gene variants will eventually guide antihyperlipidemic intervention. In this review, we discuss methodological approaches to discover genetic markers predictive of class-wide and drug-specific statin efficacy and safety. Notable pharmacogenetic findings are summarized from hypothesis-free genome wide and hypothesis-led candidate gene association studies. Physiogenomic models and clinical

providers using pharmacogenetics. Patients benefit with enhanced therapeutic outcomes that could lead to more streamlined drug approaches, fewer follow-up visits, cost savings, and shorter times to achieve therapeutic outcomes. As more drug–gene pathways are discovered and use of this knowledge increases, the potential for algorithm development for medication use will occur, resulting in better patient outcomes, higher standard of care, and reflect evidence-based medicine.

Precision medicine in oncology focuses on identifying which therapies are most effective for each patient based on genetic characterization of the cancer. Traditional chemotherapy is cytotoxic and destroys all cells that are rapidly dividing. The foundation of precision medicine is targeted therapies and selecting patients who will benefit most from these therapies. One of the newest aspects of precision medicine is liquid biopsy. A liquid biopsy includes analysis of circulating tumor cells, cell-free nucleic acid, or exosomes obtained from a peripheral blood draw. These can be studied individually or in combination and collected serially, providing real-time information as a patient's cancer changes.

The scope of FDA's jurisdiction over laboratory-developed tests (LDTs), and whether FDA has such jurisdiction at all, has been a heavily debated issue over the past several years. If FDA moves forward with its guidance, or Congress takes action to reform LDT and IVD regulation, a fundamental question that needs to be answered is how to divide activities regulated by FDCA from those regulated by CLIA. In this article, we consider FDA's authority to regulate LDTs and the policy implications of regulation, and discuss an idea for a fact-driven framework to distinguish FDCA- and CLIA- activities.

Extracellular vesicles (EVs) are membranous particles found in a variety of biofluids that encapsulate molecular information from the cell, which they originate from. This rich source of information that is easily obtained can then be mined to find diagnostic biomarkers. This article explores the current biological understanding of EVs and specific methods to isolate and analyze them. A case study of a company leading the charge in using EVs in diagnostic assays is provided.

Pharmacogenomics and Precision Medicine

CLINICS IN LABORATORY MEDICINE

THE CLINICS ARE NOW AVAILABLE ONLINE!
Access your subscription at:
www.theclinics.com

Preface

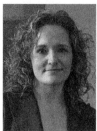 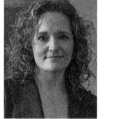

Kristen K. Reynolds, PhD   Roland Valdes Jr, PhD, DABCC, FACB
Editors

The evolution of medical practice from intuitive-to-precision approaches is driven by the accuracy of the information available for diagnostics and therapeutics. The term "precision medicine" is associated with the accuracy of a diagnosis and with understanding the molecular basis of a disease or clinical condition. Personalized medicine, on the other hand, is more narrowly defined with tailoring a therapeutic approach to an individual as compared with an average population. Both concepts are complementary and enable each other when the clinical laboratory provides actionable information. The articles in this 2016 issue of *Clinics in Laboratory Medicine* summarize updates on the rapidly evolving applications of pharmacogenetics/pharmacogenomics (PGx) used in enabling the practice of personalized, precision medicine. Previous articles in this series (2008) discussed the history of pharmacogenomics and how advanced technology transformed pharmacogenetics from a descriptive to a predictive science. Those articles also provided an extensive literature review of the genetic markers predictive of human drug response. We now update the series and present a basis for understanding the fundamental aspects of pharmacogenetics as related to its applications in anticoagulation, lipid disorders, pain management, behavioral health, and oncology. Our dive into several evolving areas, such as single-cell analysis and use of extracellular vesicles as potential diagnostic approaches, is then punctuated with questions related to what may lie in store for regulations of clinical laboratory tests in the United States and, perhaps, in international markets as well.

We begin with a review by Valdes and Yin, providing an understanding of pharmacogenetics by reviewing some key fundamental concepts in pharmacology and genetics as they apply to the discipline. The authors also briefly provide a framework for establishing the role of the clinical laboratory in this process and in enabling personalized, precision medicine. The articles that follow are enlightening and begin with an article by Maier, Duncan, and Hill that provides an update of PGx in antithrombotic therapy with pertinent clinical scenarios, including the application of evolving decision support algorithms. That article is followed by a review authored by Ruano and colleagues, on the pharmacogenetics of statin therapies and the use of decision support tools to optimize selection treatments for hypercholesterolemia. The therapeutics of managing pain has become complex and requires understanding of PGx for both therapeutic optimization and for

Clin Lab Med 36 (2016) xi–xiii
http://dx.doi.org/10.1016/j.cll.2016.06.001
0272-2712/16/$ – see front matter © 2016 Published by Elsevier Inc.

safety; hence, an article authored by Webster and Belfer address this application. Pharmacogenetics has applications in the area of behavioral health, a very confounding clinical area for pharmacotherapy selection. El-Mallakh and colleagues provide a detailed application of PGx in this important clinical practice. The economic impact of PGx testing has received much attention recently, and Reynolds, McNally, and Linder provide an in-depth look in an article focusing on the application of one specific gene complex in the economics across several clinical applications. An article by Weitendorf and Reynolds focuses on the important application of PGx testing on drug prescriptions and the role of the pharmacist in managing the efficacious distribution of medications. As for emerging developments, technological advances in clinical laboratory practice have made it possible to isolate single cells and elements called "extracellular vesicles," both found in blood. These are emerging applications that hold promise for individualizing diagnostics and personalized therapeutics. An article by Millner and Strotman focuses on techniques for separating single cells and subsequent analysis, making its way into clinical laboratory practice. A similar discussion is paralleled on extracellular vesicles by Strotman and Linder, again demonstrating emerging technologies for applications in laboratory medicine. We end with what may be a game-changer for laboratory practice by way of regulation of laboratory-developed tests beyond or replacing what is now managed by the CLIA mechanism. Thompson and Boiani explore legal arguments as to why the US Food and Drug Administration may be able to regulate clinical laboratory tests and may require FDA clearance—an interesting view of clinical legal ramifications.

This compendium of articles in *Clinics in Laboratory Medicine* is a great tool for practitioners and researchers contemplating the field of pharmacogenetics because it updates major areas of application in this evolving discipline as well as points out the strengths and weaknesses of the rapidly growing area of personalized, precision medicine. Physicians and other health professionals who want to gain more understanding of this exciting field in the clinical laboratory space will also find these articles stimulating. Finally, this selection of articles is a great tool for students anxious to learn about the science of pharmacogenetics and its current and emerging clinical applications.

Sincerely,

Kristen K. Reynolds, PhD
Department of Pathology and Laboratory Medicine
University of Louisville School of Medicine
Louisville, KY 40292, USA

VP Laboratory Operations
PGXL Laboratories
Louisville, KY 40202, USA

Roland Valdes Jr, PhD, DABCC, FACB
Departments of Pathology and Laboratory Medicine
and Biochemistry and Molecular Genetics
Chief, Clinical Chemistry and Toxicology
University of Louisville School of Medicine
Louisville, KY 40292, USA

E-mail addresses:
kreynolds@pgxlab.com (K.K. Reynolds)
roland.valdes@pgxlab.com (R. Valdes Jr)

DEDICATION

To Dr Gary K. Ackers (1939-2011), who, as professor at the University of Virginia, mentored my PhD training and inspired a rigorous scientific approach, shaping my career and personal life, to whom I remain most grateful. Roland Valdes Jr.

Fundamentals of Pharmacogenetics in Personalized, Precision Medicine

CrossMark

Roland Valdes Jr, PhD, DABCC[a,b,*], DeLu (Tyler) Yin, PhD[c]

KEYWORDS

- Pharmacogenetics • Personalized medicine • Precision medicine
- Pharmacogenomics

KEY POINTS

- Precision medicine is used as it applies to the accuracy of a diagnosis and the precision with which a diagnosis is made.
- Personalized medicine applies to a therapeutic approach tailored to optimize a therapy specific to an individual as contrasted to a group of individuals.
- Pharmacogenetics (PGx) is used to denote clinical testing of genetic variation to assess response to drugs. PGx is an integral component to both precision medicine and personalized medicine.

PERSONALIZED AND PRECISION MEDICINE

What is "precision" medicine and does it differ from "personalized" medicine? Although these 2 concepts have operationally different definitions, they complement each other in application. "Precision" medicine is used as it applies to the accuracy of a diagnosis and the precision with which a diagnosis is made. In essence, precision medicine is linked to the definition of a true disease state and to understanding pathologic mechanisms.[1] With regard to a laboratory test, the concept of "clinical validity" as defined by agencies and professional organizations is a good analogy as to how well does the test result define a condition of interest.[2]

Personalized medicine applies to a therapeutic approach tailored to optimize a therapy specific to an individual as contrasted to a group of individuals.[1] The concept

[a] Department of Pathology and Laboratory Medicine, University of Louisville School of Medicine, MDR Building, Room 222, 511 South Floyd Street, Louisville, KY 40202, USA; [b] Department of Biochemistry and Molecular Genetics, University of Louisville School of Medicine, HSC-A Building, Louisville, KY 40202, USA; [c] Department of Pathology and Laboratory Medicine, University of Louisville School of Medicine, MDR Building, Room 218, 511 South Floyd Street, Louisville, KY 40202, USA
* Corresponding author. Department of Pathology and Laboratory Medicine, University of Louisville School of Medicine, MDR Building, Room 222, 511 South Floyd Street, Louisville, KY 40202.
E-mail address: roland.valdes@louisville.edu

Clin Lab Med 36 (2016) 447–459
http://dx.doi.org/10.1016/j.cll.2016.05.006
0272-2712/16/$ – see front matter © 2016 Elsevier Inc. All rights reserved.

of a personalized approach to therapy has been used since the inception of modern medical practice. Examples are in the selection of blood products for transfusions and of matched tissues for transplantation, both based on biochemical information specific to the donor and recipient. Advances in technologies have increased the precision with which we can tailor a specific therapy to a particular individual. These advances have created emphasis on the concepts of personalized and precision medicine and, although they have different definitions, they enable each other in practice. One application that has greatly improved the personalization of therapeutics is the introduction of pharmacogenetics (PGx) as a subdiscipline in laboratory medicine. To appreciate this laboratory discipline it is important to understand basic elements of pharmacology applied to clinical practice.

OVERVIEW OF THERAPEUTIC DRUG MONITORING, PHARMACOLOGY, AND PHARMACOGENETICS

Therapeutic drug monitoring (TDM), or more recently referred to as therapeutic drug management, involves using measured serum drug concentrations along with pharmacokinetic (PK) and pharmacodynamic (PD) principles to optimize a patient's response to drug therapy. The response to drug concentrations may be therapeutic, subtherapeutic, or toxic, and these depend on considerations involving both PK and PD. The aim is to optimize therapeutic response by maintaining serum drug concentrations within a therapeutic range (the concentration at which the drug maximizes effectiveness and minimizes toxicity). TDM is applied most effectively to a small number of drugs with a narrow range of safe and effective serum drug concentrations. **Fig. 1** shows the conceptual relationship among dose rate, PK, serum drug concentration, and pharmacologic response.[3] The health care provider will determine the dose and frequency of drug administration, typically based on the drug's known bioavailability and clearance rate, which will result in steady-state serum concentrations that provide the expected therapeutic response. Examples of drugs that typically are monitored using TDM principles are amikacin, amitriptyline, carbamazepine, cyclosporine, digoxin, gentamicin, imipramine, lidocaine, lithium, methotrexate, nortriptyline, phenytoin, theophylline, tobramycin, valproic acid, and vancomycin, among others.

Pharmacology is the study of drugs and how the function of living tissues and organisms is modified by the effect of drugs and other chemical substances. Historically, knowledge of pharmacologic responses to drugs has been based on average population responses. Gene-based technologies provide information specific to an individual's drug

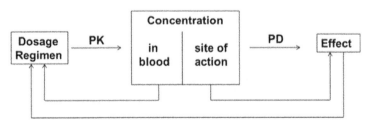

Fig. 1. Conceptual relationship between PK and PD. PK relates to the effect of the body on the drug and principally includes bioavailability, distribution, and clearance. PD relates to drug concentration and receptor availability. The net effect is dependent on both PK and PD. (*Adapted from* Linder MW, Valdes R Jr. Pharmacogenetics: fundamentals and applications. Therapeutic drug monitoring and toxicology. vol. 20(1). Washington, DC: AACC; 1999. p. 9–17; and Burtis, et al. Tietz textbook of clinical chemistry. Philadelphia: W.B. Saunders; 1999.)

response characteristics. Two fundamental principles driving individualizing drug response are PK and PD (see **Fig. 1**).[4] Understanding these 2 concepts is important, because they form the basis for how PGx leads to a focused personalized medicine approach to pharmacotherapy.

PK describes the rates of processing and transport of drugs by a living organism, including the rates of absorption, distribution, metabolism, and excretion commonly referred to by the acronym ADME.[4] Many biological, physiologic, and physicochemical factors influence the transfer processes of drugs in the body and influence the overall rate and extent of ADME. PK analysis is used to determine the dose of a drug required to provide the steady-state concentration of the medicine needed to achieve the required therapeutic response and is one key element for establishing a rational design of an individualized dosage regimen. The main objectives are to maintain an optimum drug concentration at the receptor site, to produce the desired therapeutic response for a specific period, and to minimize any adverse or toxic effects of the drug. The relationship between the dose of a drug and the subsequent concentration of the drug in blood[5] determines the concentration-time curve, or area under the curve (AUC), of a drug in blood as shown in **Fig. 2A**.[6] The average steady-state concentration of a drug ($C_{avg\ ss}$) is maintained by dose rate, bioavailability (f), and clearance (Cl) of the drug. The catalytic activity of drug-metabolizing enzymes (DMEs) is the principal determinant of the drug extraction ratio (ER), which is a measure of the fraction of drug cleared from circulation as it passes through whichever organ is involved in its metabolism.[4] The extraction ratio is a component of bioavailability and clearance of the drug (for more detail see **Fig. 2** in Ref.[7]).

PD describes the effect of the drug on the body and is based on principles founded on the receptor occupancy theory,[4] which is central to understanding drug action. This process begins with the action of a drug on the target cells, as shown in **Fig. 2B**, and is affected by the number and affinity of receptors, as well as the drug concentration at the receptor site. This underlies the importance of achieving a sustained steady-state effective concentration of drugs in the fluids bathing the receptors (eg, intracellular fluid, blood, cerebrospinal fluid). The relationship between the blood concentration of a drug and the response caused by that drug is shown in **Fig. 3**.[6] **Fig. 3A**

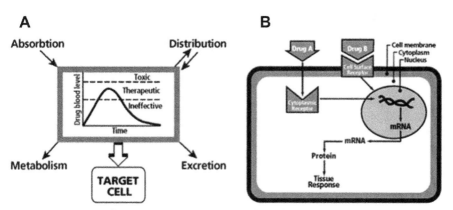

Fig. 2. Relationship of elements regulating PK and PD. (*A*) AUC for a drug dose and the elements controlling the shape and magnitude of the curve, typically absorption, distribution, metabolism, and excretion. (*B*) Interaction of a drug with a cell surface receptor or a cytoplasmic receptor. (*From* Weber W. Human drug response. In: Bobrow M, Harper PS, Scriver C, et al, editors. Pharmacogenetics. New York: Oxford University Press; 1997. By permission of Oxford University Press, USA.)

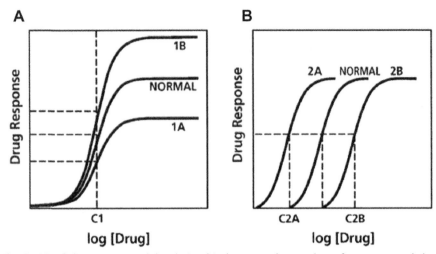

Fig. 3. PD of drug response. (*A*) Relationship between the number of receptors and drug response, where 1A is a low number, and 1B is a high number of receptors. (*B*) Relationship of drug response to affinity of receptors, where 2A is a high-affinity receptor, and 2B is low affinity. The 50% effective drug concentration C2A is lower for a high-affinity receptor compared with concentration C2B. (*From* Weber W. Human drug response. In: Bobrow M, Harper PS, Scriver C, et al, editors. Pharamcogenetics. New York: Oxford University Press; 1997. By permission of Oxford University Press, USA.)

depicts the number of available receptors, and **Fig. 3**B depicts the affinity of the receptors. Genetic contributions are responsible for both scenarios. Genetic variants (ie, polymorphisms) in the promoter region of a gene responsible for expressing the receptor protein may reduce the number of receptors, whereas genetic variants in the coding region may affect the affinity of the receptors.[5]

PHARMACOGENETICS IS FUNDAMENTAL TO PHARMACOTHERAPEUTICS

What does PGx information add to personalized, precision medicine? Basically, applied PGx allows one to more comprehensively determine, a priori, the selection of an appropriate medicine as well as the dosing optimal to an individual based on that individual's genetic characteristics. The application of TDM using measurements of drug concentrations in blood, albeit very useful, has limitations based on the amount of information it provides. To appreciate the limitation, we need to understand the biochemical basis of PK and PD. These 2 processes are based on the actions of 3 types of proteins that together comprise the "state" of an individual's drug response profile: proteins that metabolize drugs, proteins that transport drugs, and proteins as receptors of the drugs (**Fig. 4**). Monitoring blood concentrations does provide

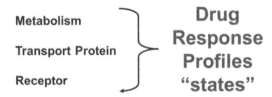

Fig. 4. The Drug Response Profile concept predicted by gene-based components is based on individualized therapeutic approaches driven by combining genotypes into individual "response states."

practical "net" information as to bioavailability, metabolism, transport, and excretion. However, the receptor protein status is not directly available by measuring concentration of drug in blood and neither does TDM allow (because it is performed after dosing) a priori information for predicting dosing parameters or selection of the drug itself in any one individual. Predicting dosing and drug function has advantages in minimizing potential toxicity, reducing adjustments in dosing, optimizing drug efficacy,[8] and, among other logistical health care advantages, avoiding drug-drug interactions.[9]

OVERVIEW OF PHARMACOGENETICS
Introduction to Genetic Concepts

A gene is a linear sequence of nucleotides; these nucleotides are joined together in sequence by means of a phosphodiester bond between the 50 and 30 carbons of the deoxyribose moiety of the nucleotide. Genes consist of a long strand of DNA containing a promoter that controls the activity of a gene and its coding and noncoding sequences. The coding sequence determines what protein the gene produces, whereas noncoding sequences can regulate the conditions of gene expression. A gene is the basic physical and functional unit of heredity; the proper scientific term for this functional unit is allele. Alleles are forms of the same gene with differences in their sequence of DNA bases. These differences contribute to each person's unique physical features and phenotypes. When a gene contains the proper elements, the coding and noncoding sequences are copied by transcription, producing an mRNA copy of the gene's information.[10] This mRNA then can direct the synthesis of the protein by means of the genetic code.[10]

Genetic Polymorphism in Pharmacogenetics

Genetic polymorphism occurs as structural changes, including nucleotide substitution, complete gene deletion, gene duplication, and genetic translocation where portions of similar genes are combined creating a new gene hybrid. The most common form of genetic polymorphism is a single nucleotide polymorphism (SNP) in which the nucleotide sequence at one specific position is changed by substitution, translocation, insertion, or deletion.[11] Each of these changes in the gene structure introduces a variant form of the gene into the population gene pool and is designated an allele of the original gene.[11] An allele is an inherited gene that is present in each nucleated cell of the body. Because of the diploid structure of the human genome, each cell carries 2 copies of each gene. Two copies of the same allele yield a homozygous genotype and any combination of 2 different alleles yields a heterozygous genotype.

The various types of genetic polymorphism are generally classified by their resulting influence on protein expression (eg, metabolizing enzyme, transport proteins, or drug receptor) or ultimate phenotype. Genetic polymorphism resulting in gene deletion invariably leads to loss of function and no production of the gene product. In contrast, gene duplication and multiduplication most commonly leads to increased expression of the gene product and a hyperactivity phenotype.[11] An exception to this is duplication of an allele that includes additional structural variation leading to loss of function. Genetic translocation typically yields a nonfunctional gene. SNPs can result in various changes in the expressed protein function depending on where the polymorphism occurs in the overall gene structure. SNPs in the regulatory domain may influence gene regulation.[11] SNPs in the coding exons only influence function if there is a resulting amino acid change that alters the protein function.[11] SNPs within the intron regions are typically silent unless the SNP alters a nucleotide critical for splicing of the RNA during maturation, which typically leads to loss or decrease in protein function.[11] One important example is the CYP2D6 enzyme system, known to metabolize many of the most widely prescribed drugs in the United States for depression, cardiovascular disease, schizophrenia, attention-deficit/hyperactivity disorder, prevention of nausea and vomiting for patients undergoing cancer chemotherapy, and symptoms of allergies and colds.[12–15] As such, we focus our discussion on the cytochrome P450 proteins, as they are the major proteins involved in the metabolism phase of PGx. The fundamentals are similar in principle for the transport proteins as well as the drug receptor proteins.

EXAMPLE OF CYTOCHROME P450 AND DRUG METABOLISM

In relation to pharmacology, cytochrome P450s (CYPs) are a family of heme-containing enzymes that catalyze the conversion of lipophilic substances into hydrophilic molecules that can then be excreted by the kidneys into the urine.[5] They represent a major part of the body's powerful detoxification systems. The CYP system metabolizes endogenous and exogenous substrates through various reactions, including epoxidation, N-dealkylation, O-dealkylation, S-oxidation, hydroxylation, and others.[16] Exogenous substances (products ingested or absorbed) include not only pharmaceutical compounds given as therapeutic drugs, but also foodstuffs, dietary components, occupational pollutants, and industrial chemicals.[5] As a group, the CYP450 enzymes often are referred to as DMEs. The metabolic process generally is described as having 2 phases, based on the nature of the transformation. Phase 1 involves an oxidative process, whereas phase 2 metabolism is generally conjugative.[5] The CYP mixed-function mono-oxygenase system is probably the most important element of phase 1 metabolism in mammals.[17] Importantly, more than half of all drugs are cleared primarily by the CYP system.[5]

The CYP system is a gene family found at multiple chromosome loci, each with tandem arrays of genes, and each gene with substantial polymorphism.[5] This system is an illustration of gene expansion, multigene families, and allelic functional variation. Genomics as a discipline has supplied a rich resource of gene mapping data and the individual variants in each gene at the SNP and chromosome locus levels. The CYP isoforms now known in people, along with the hundreds of genetic variations, have produced a large set of biomarkers believed to be predictive of susceptibility to specific toxins.[5] The fact that the pharmaceutical industry routinely includes an assessment of the main metabolic pathways of a candidate drug to derive clinical pharmacologic correlations is indicative of the importance of this knowledge.[5] Additionally, certain CYP alleles also can be markers of disease susceptibility and some are known to be implicated in detoxification or activation of environmental toxins associated with cancer risk.[11,18]

The CYP Nomenclature Committee (www.cypalleles.ki.se) has defined the nomenclature used to categorize the variant alleles of the CYP enzyme system. In general, the descriptors rely on the hierarchy of the genetic structures involved in the construction of the enzymes. **Fig. 5** describes the common basis for CYP nomenclature.[4,19] For most CYP genes, in which genetic polymorphism has been characterized, the most common sequence and that which is active, is denoted by the gene abbreviation followed by an asterisk and the number 1. This allele then serves as the reference sequence to which all other alleles of that gene are compared.[11] Of the CYP enzymes described to date, those most closely related to clinical applications through PGx testing are the 2D6, 2C9, and 2C19 enzymes, which play a role in the metabolism of more than 30% of all prescription drugs.[15,20] Factors such as high prevalence of variants in human populations and a wide range of therapeutics metabolized by these enzymes render them among the most relevant DMEs for PGx diagnostics.[5]

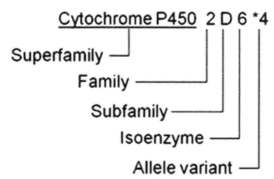

Fig. 5. Nomenclature system for designating enzymes and alleles of cytochrome P450. (*From* Linder MW, Valdes R Jr. Pharmacogenetics: fundamentals and applications. Therapeutic drug monitoring and toxicology. vol. 20(1). Washington, DC: AACC; 1999. p. 11; with permission.)

CYP2D6 polymorphisms have different prevalence and effects among population subgroups. For example, CYP2D6 polymorphisms associated with slow drug metabolism are found in approximately 5% to 10% of whites and 1% to 3% of Hispanic, African American, and Asian American individuals.[15]

CLINICAL APPLICATIONS OF PHARMACOGENETICS

The terms pharmacogenomics and pharmacogenetics have been used interchangeably.[21] PGx is generally used to denote clinical testing of genetic variation to assess response to drugs, whereas pharmacogenomics refers to the broader application of genomic technologies to the study of variations of DNA and RNA characteristics related to drug response.[22,23] The clinical utility of PGx is in the ability to predict the most appropriate dosing of a medicine (usually based on metabolic information) and/or the selection of a particular medicine for a given individual (usually based on metabolism or receptor status).[24] Most alleles encoding DMEs are within a somatic chromosome and are inherited in a non–sex-linked Mendelian fashion.[24] On the basis of observed phenotyping data, such as metabolic ratios of drug components in blood and urine, a reasonable separation can be demonstrated between extensive metabolizers (normal metabolizers), rapid metabolizers (generally referred to as ultrarapid), and poor metabolizers in their ability to biotransform specific medications. The differences between these phenotypes are explained in **Box 1**.[25] This nomenclature has been challenged as not being sufficiently descriptive and requiring modification; however, it persists.[5]

One anticipated clinical outcome of PGx diagnostics is in reducing adverse drug reactions (ADRs). ADRs are a consequence of nearly 3 million incorrect or ineffective drug prescriptions annually[15] and PGx testing holds promise to help prescribe drugs and dosages in ways that fit individual patient responses and reduce the number of ADRs.[15,26]

Another important application of PGx is in helping to reduce polypharmacy. Polypharmacy is the use of multiple medications and is growing at an alarming rate with reports documenting a range of 5 to 17 prescriptions being used on average by individuals older than 69 years.[27] The health care consequences range from drug-drug interactions, adverse drug events, prescribing cascades, chronic dependence, and hospitalizations, all of which have significant health and economic consequences. PGx profiles, drug-drug interaction information, and advance health

---

Box 1
Phenotypic categories as determined by pharmacogenetic testing for cytochrome P450 enzymes

Ultraextensive metabolizers (UM): may require an increased dosage because of higher than normal rates of drug metabolism. Simultaneously treating with medication that inhibits metabolism also has proven effective. Genotypes consistent with UM phenotype include 3 or more active genes producing the drug-metabolizing enzyme and therefore have increased metabolic capacity.

Extensive metabolizers (EM): represent the norm for metabolic capacity. Genotypes consistent with the EM phenotype include 2 active forms of the gene producing the drug-metabolizing enzyme and therefore possess the full complement of drug-metabolizing capacity. Generally, EMs can be administered drugs, which are substrates of the enzyme following standard dosing practices.

Intermediate metabolizers (IM): may require lower than average drug dosages for optimal therapeutic response. In addition, multiple drug therapy should be monitored closely.

Poor metabolizers (PM): are at increased risk of drug-induced adverse effects because of diminished drug elimination (accumulation) or lack of therapeutic effect resulting from failure to generate the active form of the drug. Genotypes consistent with the PM phenotype are those with no active genes producing the drug-metabolizing enzyme. These individuals have a deficiency in drug metabolism.

Data from Valdes R Jr, Payne D, Linder M, et al. Laboratory analysis and application of pharmacogenetics to clinical practice. Washington, DC: National Academy of Biochemistry; 2010. Available at: https://www.aacc.org/~/media/practice-guidelines/pharmacogenetics/pgx_guidelines.pdf?la=en.

---

informatics technology can be combined to prevent or reduce the overuse of multiple medications and avoid complications.[28]

Another benefit of PGx testing is improving the productivity of new drug pipelines.[15,29] The use of PGx in clinical trial design and patient accrual could lead to reductions in the time needed to develop a drug from 10 to 12 years to perhaps as little as 3 to 5 years.[15] The ability to stratify patient groups using genomic biomarkers should enable selection of treatment or causative effects that otherwise would have been diluted in more heterogeneous populations. In addition to these applications, and from a pharmacotherapeutic perspective, the use of PGx information may enable development of drugs tailored for patients who have rare or orphan conditions and other underserved patient groups.[15,29]

Central to the clinical applications discussed previously is deciding when in the therapeutic-decision pathway to use the PGx information. The ability to more precisely predict drug response a priori to selection of drug and/or dosing can now change therapeutic paradigms. One schema is shown in **Fig. 6**.[30]

An example to emphasize the basis and potential of applying PGx information to predict drug dosing and timing and its impact is shown in **Fig. 7**. It illustrates the power of how PGx variants predict both drug accumulation as well as time to reach a steady-state drug concentration in blood, both dependent on genetic variant.[31]

Clinical application of PGx has the potential to improve treatments for chronic diseases that pose the greatest morbidity and cost burden for the United States and other developed nations. One example is in oncology therapeutics with the drug tamoxifen[32] used to treat breast cancer. Tamoxifen is an inactive prodrug that must be metabolized by CYP2D6 into its more potent metabolite, endoxifen, to maximize its effect. Knowing a patient's CYP2D6 metabolic status can be used to predict the success of tamoxifen therapy.[33]

The explanatory (old) role of
pharmacogenetics:

The predictive (new) role of
pharmacogenetics:

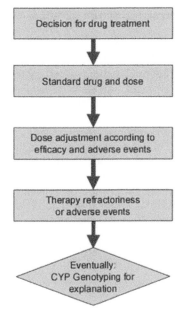

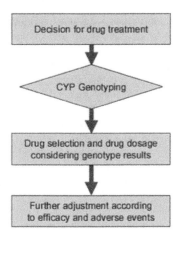

Fig. 6. New model (do we explain or predict?). The diamond box indicates the location of the PGx information in the decision making process. (*From* Brockmöller J, Kirchheiner J, Meisel C, Roots I. Pharmacogenetic diagnostics of cytochrome P450 polymorphisms in clinical drug development and in drug treatment. Pharmacogenomics 2000;1(2):137; with permission.)

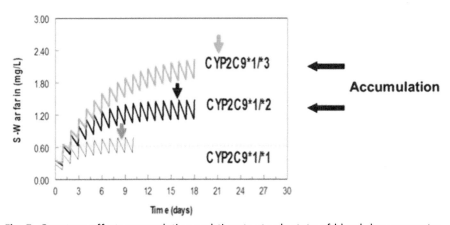

Fig. 7. Genotype affects accumulation and time to steady state of blood drug concentrations. Example of warfarin concentrations for 3 genotypes with genetic variants of CYP2C9. Note the time to reach steady state (*vertical arrows*) and accumulated concentration of drug (*horizontal arrows*) are genotype variant-dependent. (*From* Linder MW, Looney S, Adams JE, et al. Warfarin dose adjustments based on CYP2C9 genetic polymorphisms. J Thromb Thrombolysis 2002;14(3):231; with permission.)

Other examples of costly chronic diseases are those involving behavioral health, such as schizophrenia[34] and depression.[35] Treatments of these conditions involve considerable medication trial-and-error approaches and have high health care cost consequences. The use of PGx-guided treatments has shown to reduce costs as well as increase treatment efficiencies.[34–36]

Companion diagnostics is another application of PGx. Companion diagnostics refers to developing biological markers associated with specific drugs to determine efficacy and/or selection for optimum use. This is now recommended by the Food and Drug Administration (FDA) for drugs in development[37] and is becoming standard of care, particularly in oncology. Some examples are listed in **Table 1**.

Progress in the use of PGX is accelerating, yet relevant regulatory agencies are just catching up. Despite current attention on a small number of recent molecular break-throughs, which represents the tip of the iceberg, much of the potential health benefit of PGx resides in some of the longer-standing, more widely used products. Most ADRs, including many that are likely to be influenced by genotype, arise with use of older drugs. An FDA Web site documents more than 140 drugs having a genetic component to their efficacy.[38] Although much of the valuable information involving PGx available today remains to be put to use,[39] evidence strongly indicates that interindividual genetic variations result in variation in drug transporters, DMEs, and drug targets, all contributing to differences in how people respond to the same medications.

THE CLINICAL LABORATORY AS CATALYST

The clinical laboratory is the principal vehicle for providing PGx testing services to the medical community.[40] These services include providing access to testing, selecting appropriate testing profiles and, among other responsibilities, providing the evidence required to formulate decisions on medical applications.[40] In recent years, the number of clinical laboratories providing PGx testing services have blossomed. According to the 2015 survey from the College of American Pathologists, 135 laboratories partici-pated in the PGX-B mailing list alone.[41] The use of gene-based information to stratify patients, preferably before they are prescribed medication requires integration of test results with advanced informatics technology. Methods involving algorithms able to translate the genetic information inherent in the marker (eg, SNP variants in genes for metabolic enzymes or receptors) into a quantifiable and reliable dosing or drug selection schema are taking hold. One example is demonstrated by Linder and col-leagues[31] with an algorithm for dosing the anticoagulant warfarin. This is only one example and others have been reported, including those involving PGxs profiles linked to drug-drug interaction databases.[42–48] Although the future of PGx in the clinical laboratory is still in its infancy, it has enormous possibilities.[24,49–51] This speaks to the value of the clinical laboratory as a catalyst in enabling personalized, precision medicine.

Table 1
KRAS codes for a GTPase; BRAF codes for Serine/threonine-protein kinase; ALK fusion codes for a lymphoma kinase

Gene Mutation	Drug(s) Selection	Clinical Condition
KRAS	Vectibix (panitumumab) Erbitux (cetuximab)	Colon and lung cancers
BRAF	Zelboraf (Vemurafenib)	Melanoma
ALK	Xalkori (crizotinib)	Non–small cell lung cancers

REFERENCES

1. Christensen CM, Grossman JH, Hwang J. The innovator's prescription: a disruptive solution for health care. New York: McGraw-Hill; 2009.
2. Evans BJ, Burke W, Jarvik GP. The FDA and genomic tests—getting regulation right. N Engl J Med 2015;372(23):2258–64.
3. Burtis CA, Ashwood ER, Tietz NW. Tietz textbook of clinical chemistry. Philadelphia: W.B. Saunders; 1999.
4. Linder MW, Valdes R Jr. Fundamentals of pharmacogenetics. Washington, DC: AACC Press; 2006.
5. Valdes R Jr, Payne DA, Linder MW. Laboratory analysis and application of pharmacogenetics to clinical practice. National Academy of Clinical Biochemistry. Available at: https://www.aacc.org/~/media/practice-guidelines/pharmacogenetics/pgx_guidelines.pdf?la=en. Accessed February 15, 2015.
6. Weber W. Human drug response. New York: Oxford University Press; 1997.
7. Al-Ghoul M, Valdes R Jr. Fundamentals of pharmacology and applications in pharmacogenetics. Philadelphia: Elsevier Saunders; 2008.
8. Daughton CG, Ruhoy IS. Lower-dose prescribing: minimizing "side effects" of pharmaceuticals on society and the environment. Sci Total Environ 2013;443:324–37.
9. Murray M. Role of CYP pharmacogenetics and drug-drug interactions in the efficacy and safety of atypical and other antipsychotic agents. J Pharm Pharmacol 2006;58(7):871–85.
10. Gerstein MB, Bruce C, Rozowsky JS, et al. What is a gene, post-ENCODE? History and updated definition. Genome Res 2007;17(6):669–81.
11. Linder MW, Valdes R Jr. Genetic mechanisms for variability in drug response and toxicity. J Anal Toxicol 2001;25(5):405–13.
12. Johnson JA, Cavallari LH. Cardiovascular pharmacogenomics. Exp Physiol 2005;90(3):283–9.
13. Agúndez JAG, Gallardo L, Ledesma MC, et al. Functionally active duplications of the CYP2D6 gene are more prevalent among larynx and lung cancer patients. Oncology 2001;61(1):59–63.
14. Johnson JA, Humma LM. Pharmacogenetics of cardiovascular drugs. Brief Funct Genomics 2002;1(1):66–79.
15. Tuckson RV, Au SM, Berry CE, et al. Realizing the promise of pharmacogenomics: opportunities and challenges. Biotechnol Rep 2007;26(3):261–91.
16. Wilkinson GR. Drug metabolism and variability among patients in drug response. New Engl J Med 2005;352(21):2211–21.
17. de Leon J, Armstrong SC, Cozza KL. Clinical guidelines for psychiatrists for the use of pharmacogenetic testing for CYP450 2D6 and CYP450 2C19. Psychosomatics 2006;47(1):75–85.
18. Feigelson HS, McKean-Cowdin R, Coetzee GA, et al. Building a multigenic model of breast cancer susceptibility: CYP17 and HSD17B1 are two important candidates. Cancer Res 2001;61(2):785–9.
19. Nelson DR, Kamataki T, Waxman DJ, et al. The P450 superfamily: update on new sequences, gene mapping, accession numbers, early trivial names of enzymes, and nomenclature. DNA Cell Biol 1993;12(1):1–51.
20. Phillips KA, Van Bebber SL. Measuring the value of pharmacogenomics. Nat Rev Drug Discov 2005;4(6):500–9.
21. Khoury MJ. Genetics and genomics in practice: the continuum from genetic disease to genetic information in health and disease. Genet Med 2003;5(4):261–8.

22. Sikka R, Magauran B, Ulrich A, et al. Bench to bedside: pharmacogenomics, adverse drug interactions, and the cytochrome P450 system. Acad Emerg Med 2005;12(12):1227–35.
23. Weinshilboum R, Wang L. Pharmacogenomics: bench to bedside. Nat Rev Drug Discov 2004;3(9):739–48.
24. Linder MW, Valdes R Jr. Fundamentals and applications of pharmacogenetics for the clinical laboratory. Ann Clin Lab Sci 1999;29(2):140–9.
25. Linder MW, Prough RA, Valdes R Jr. Pharmacogenetics: a laboratory tool for optimizing therapeutic efficiency. Clin Chem 1997;43(2):254–66.
26. Hopkins MM, Ibarreta D, Gaisser S, et al. Putting pharmacogenetics into practice. Nat Biotechnol 2006;24(4):403–10.
27. Steinman MA, Seth Landefeld C, Rosenthal GE, et al. Polypharmacy and prescribing quality in older people. J Am Geriatr Soc 2006;54(10):1516–23.
28. Reynolds KK , Weitendorf F, Linder MW. Correlation of pharmacogenetic results with patient medication regimens: a pilot study for reporting gene-drug and drug-drug interactions with pharmacy support. Presented at the Association for Molecular Pathology Annual Meeting. National Harbor, MD, October 2014.
29. Schmedders M, van Aken J, Feuerstein G, et al. Individualized pharmacogenetic therapy: a critical analysis. Community Genet 2003;6(2):114–9.
30. Brockmöller J, Kirchheiner J, Meisel C, et al. Pharmacogenetic diagnostics of cytochrome P450 polymorphisms in clinical drug development and in drug treatment. Pharmacogenomics 2000;1(2):125–51.
31. Linder MW, Looney S, Adams JE 3rd, et al. Warfarin dose adjustments based on CYP2C9 genetic polymorphisms. J Thromb Thrombolysis 2002;14(3):227–32.
32. Goetz MP, Kamal A, Ames MM. Tamoxifen pharmacogenomics: the role of CYP2D6 as a predictor of drug response. Clin Pharmacol Ther 2008;83(1):160–6.
33. Saladores P, Murdter T, Eccles D, et al. Tamoxifen metabolism predicts drug concentrations and outcome in premenopausal patients with early breast cancer. Pharmacogenomics J 2015;15(1):84–94.
34. Herbild L, Andersen SE, Werge T, et al. Does pharmacogenetic testing for CYP450 2D6 and 2C19 among patients with diagnoses within the schizophrenic spectrum reduce treatment costs? Basic Clin Pharmacol Toxicol 2013;113(4): 266–72.
35. Winner J, Allen JD, Altar CA, et al. Psychiatric pharmacogenomics predicts health resource utilization of outpatients with anxiety and depression. Transl Psychiatry 2013;3:e242.
36. Chou WH, Yan FX, de Leon J, et al. Extension of a pilot study: impact from the cytochrome P450 2D6 polymorphism on outcome and costs associated with severe mental illness. J Clin Psychopharmacol 2000;20(2):246–51.
37. Maliepaard M, Nofziger C, Papaluca M, et al. Pharmacogenetics in the evaluation of new drugs: a multiregional regulatory perspective. Nat Rev Drug Discov 2013; 12(2):103–15.
38. Food and Drug Administration. Table of pharmacogenomic biomarkers in drug labeling. Food and Drug Administration. Available at: http://www.fda.gov/Drugs/ScienceResearch/ResearchAreas/Pharmacogenetics/ucm083378.htm. Accessed February 15, 2015.
39. Haga SB, Mills R, Moaddeb J. Pharmacogenetic information for patients on drug labels. Pharmgenomics Pers Med 2014;7:297–305.
40. Linder MW, Valdes R Jr. Pharmacogenetics in the practice of laboratory medicine. Mol Diagn 1999;4(4):365–79.
41. CAP Participant Summary. PGXB Inc; 2015. p. 6.

42. Schelleman H, Chen J, Chen Z, et al. Dosing algorithms to predict warfarin maintenance dose in Caucasians and African Americans. Clin Pharmacol Ther 2008; 84(3):332–9.
43. Klein TE, Altman RB, Eriksson N, et al. Estimation of the warfarin dose with clinical and pharmacogenetic data. N Engl J Med 2009;360(8):753–64.
44. Millican EA, Lenzini PA, Milligan PE, et al. Genetic-based dosing in orthopedic patients beginning warfarin therapy. Blood 2007;110(5):1511–5.
45. Hillman MA, Wilke RA, Yale SH, et al. A prospective, randomized pilot trial of model-based warfarin dose initiation using CYP2C9 genotype and clinical data. Clin Med Res 2005;3(3):137–45.
46. Gage BF, Eby C, Johnson JA, et al. Use of pharmacogenetic and clinical factors to predict the therapeutic dose of warfarin. Clin Pharmacol Ther 2008;84(3): 326–31.
47. Carlquist JF, Anderson JL. Using pharmacogenetics in real time to guide warfarin initiation: a clinician update. Circulation 2011;124(23):2554–9.
48. Tham LS, Goh BC, Nafziger A, et al. A warfarin-dosing model in Asians that uses single-nucleotide polymorphisms in vitamin K epoxide reductase complex and cytochrome P450 2C9. Clin Pharmacol Ther 2006;80(4):346–55.
49. Valdes R Jr, Linder MW. Fine-tuning pharmacogenetics: paradigm for linking laboratory results to clinical action. Clin Chem 2004;50(9):1498–9.
50. Valdes R Jr, Linder MW, Jortani SA. What is next in pharmacogenomics? Translating it to clinical practice. Pharmacogenomics 2003;4(4):499–505.
51. Linder MW, Valdes R Jr. Pharmacogenetics: fundamentals and applications. Therapeutic drug monitoring and toxicology, vol. 20(1). Washington, DC: AACC; 1999. p. 9–17.

Pharmacogenetics in Oral Antithrombotic Therapy

Cheryl L. Maier, MD, PhD*, Alexander Duncan, MD, Charles E. Hill, MD, PhD

KEYWORDS

- Pharmacogenetics • Pharmacogenomics • Antithrombotic • Antiplatelet
- Anticoagulant • Personalized medicine

KEY POINTS

- Vitamin K antagonists (VKA) are affected by *CYP2C9* and *VKORC1* polymorphisms that lead to variable dose responses.
- New direct oral anticoagulants (DOAC) are not affected by *CYP2C9* and *VKORC1* polymorphisms; however, DOAC may be affected by other genes related to their metabolism.
- Aspirin response is multifactorial, and studies have failed to identify genetic determinants of aspirin nonresponse.
- *CYP2C19* polymorphisms cause variable responses to clopidogrel, which can result in subtherapeutic platelet inhibition; however, additional undetermined genetic factors may also be involved.
- Newer P2Y12 inhibitors prasugrel and ticagrelor are not affected by *CYP2C19* and seem less susceptible to genetic variation than clopidogrel, although further study is needed.

INTRODUCTION

The human body maintains a delicate balance between bleeding and clotting, and optimal antithrombotic therapy aims to modulate hemostasis while avoiding either thrombosis or hemorrhage. Two predominant classes of antithrombotic drugs are the anticoagulant agents, which are generally used to prevent and treat venous thromboembolism (VTE) like pulmonary embolism and deep vein thrombosis, and the antiplatelet agents, which are generally used to prevent and treat arterial clots involved in conditions like myocardial infarction (MI) and thromboembolic stroke. Interindividual variability in drug response complicates antithrombotic therapy, with subtherapeutic levels reducing the effectiveness and supratherapeutic levels increasing the risk of bleeding. Such variability is influenced by clinical factors like age, sex, renal and

The authors have nothing to disclose.
Department of Pathology and Laboratory Medicine, Emory University Hospital, Emory University School of Medicine, 1364 Clifton Road Northeast, Atlanta, GA 30322, USA
* Corresponding author.
E-mail address: cheryl.maier@emory.edu

Clin Lab Med 36 (2016) 461–472
http://dx.doi.org/10.1016/j.cll.2016.05.002
0272-2712/16/$ – see front matter © 2016 Elsevier Inc. All rights reserved.

labmed.theclinics.com

hepatic function, metabolic disorders like diabetes, and concomitant medications, and also by genetic factors that impact drug bioavailability and therapeutic targets.

Pharmacogenetics is a relatively new but promising field that studies how variation in individual genes affects responses to drugs.[1] Genetic polymorphisms can alter pharmacologic responses by influencing drug absorption, distribution, and metabolism, and by altering drug targets.[2] Understanding the genetic factors that modulate therapeutic response may allow clinicians to optimize drug efficacy while minimizing adverse events, a key consideration in antithrombotic therapy. Pharmacogenetics has revealed important genetic determinants that affect patients' responses to warfarin and clopidogrel, drugs that are cornerstones of antithrombotic therapy. However, the clinical utility of genetic testing remains controversial. Several novel antithrombotic drugs have become available that seem to be less influenced by genetic variation. Clinical trials are currently under way to further evaluate any genetic influence on the response to these new oral antithrombotics.

Recent advances in genomic technology coupled with the development of new classes of antithrombotic drugs have made this topic a dynamic and timely area of study. This review presents an overview of pharmacogenetics related to oral antithrombotic drugs, including the well-studied agents, warfarin, aspirin, and clopidogrel, and the new agents, dabigatran, rivaroxaban, apixaban, edoxaban, prasugrel, and ticagrelor.

ANTICOAGULANTS

Anticoagulants target various portions of the coagulation cascade and are primarily used to treat and prevent thrombus formation in low shear stress environments such as in veins or fibrillating atria. The introduction of a new generation of direct oral anticoagulants (DOAC) has greatly expanded oral antithrombotic therapy, which was previously limited to vitamin K antagonists (VKA). VKA target several coagulation factors and can be difficult to manage, because they have a narrow therapeutic window, significant food and drug interactions, and high interidividual and intraindividual variability, all of which necessitate frequent laboratory monitoring. The DOAC, including the direct thrombin inhibitor dabigatran and the factor Xa inhibitors rivaroxaban, apixaban, and edoxaban, target 1 specific coagulation factor and do not require routine coagulation monitoring. DOAC are at least as effective as VKA in the prevention and treatment of thromboemolic events and seem to be more convenient, with large therapeutic windows and less interindividual and intraindividual variability. Still, the major risk of DOAC therapy is bleeding and whether pharmacogenetics can mitigate this risk requires further investigation.

Vitamin K Antagonists

VKA include the coumarin derivatives warfarin, phenprocoumon, and acenocoumarol, and the indedione derivative fluindione. Warfarin remains the most prescribed oral anticoagulant worldwide, especially in North America and the UK, although the other VKA are commonly used throughout Europe.[3] Individual warfarin therapy response is monitored using the international normalized ratio of the prothrombin time to determine the degree of anticoagulation and to guide dose adjustments, with the ultimate goal of maximizing the time within the therapeutic range and, thereby, clinical outcome.

Warfarin is metabolized in the liver by CYP450 enzymes including CYP2C9, which converts the active drug into inactive metabolites, and polymorphisms in *CYP2C9* can lead to high variations in dose response.[4,5] The *CYP2C9*2* variant is about 12%

as efficient as the wild-type enzyme, and the *CYP2C9*3* variant has less than 5% wild-type activity; therefore, both are associated with lower dose requirements for reaching a target international normalized ratio.[5–7] Polymorphisms in the gene encoding vitamin K epoxide reductase complex (*VKORC1*), which converts vitamin K into its active form and is inhibited by warfarin, also account for phenotypic variability in warfarin dosing. Several single nucleotide polymorphisms (SNPs) that affect *VKORC1* expression are associated with increased sensitivity to VKA.[8,9] Genome-wide association studies (GWAS) have suggested that *CYP2C9* and *VKORC1* polymorphisms account for approximately 40% of the variability in warfarin dosing.[10,11] Clinical factors and additional genetic determinants likely contribute to the remaining variability, which ongoing studies suggest may be of variable significance in different populations.[12]

In 2007, the US Food and Drug Administration (FDA) modified the warfarin label to reflect the potential influence of *CYP2C9* or *VKORC1* polymorphisms on dose requirements, making warfarin the only pharmacologic agent for which testing of 2 independent genetic variants is currently recommended. In 2010, the FDA further modified the label to include a pharmacogenetic-guided dosing scheme to use when initiating warfarin therapy. Genetic testing for *CYP2C9* and *VKORC1* variants is available to clinicians and used in some dosing algorithms.[13] A recent meta-analysis of ten randomized controlled trials demonstrated clinical benefit of pharmacogenetic algorithm-guided warfarin dosing as compared to standard dosing strategies.[14] Nevertheless, routine genotyping of patients before initiating therapy is not widespread and is not recommended currently by the American College of Chest Physicians.[15]

Direct Oral Anticoagulants

Some investigators have proposed that the availability of DOAC will shift the focus of pharmacogenetics in antithrombotic therapy away from warfarin altogether, although further investigation is needed to determine whether genetic polymorphisms contribute to bleeding associated with DOAC therapy.[16] The Randomized Evaluation of Long Term Anticoagulant Therapy (RE-LY) With Dabigatran Etexilate study found similar rates of major bleeding events for dabigatran and warfarin,[17] and the Prospective, Randomized, Double-Blind, Parallel-Group, Multicenter, Non-inferiority Study Comparing the Efficacy and Safety of Rivaroxaban (BAY 59-7939) With Warfarin for the Prevention of Stroke and Non-Central Nervous System Systemic Embolism in Subjects With Non-Valvular Atrial Fibrillation (ROCKET) trial showed that rivaroxaban was associated with fewer intracranial or fatal bleeds as compared with warfarin.[18] Such studies have demonstrated some interindividual variability in DOAC, and the clinical consequences and contribution of genetic polymorphisms to this variability are being investigated.

Direct thrombin inhibitor—dabigatran

Dabigatran is a reversible and direct inhibitor of thrombin (factor IIa), thereby preventing the conversion of fibrinogen to fibrin. It became clinically available for use in Europe in 2008 and in the United States in 2010.[19] Dabigatran currently has many approved indications, including prevention of stroke and systemic embolism in patients with nonvalvular atrial fibrillation, treatment of VTE after parenteral anticoagulation, and VTE prophylaxis in certain patient populations (after VTE, postoperatively). The non-pharmacologically active prodrug dabigatran etexilate is administered orally, and esterases *CES1* and *CES2* rapidly hydrolyze the prodrug in the intestine and liver to the pharmacologically active drug dabigatran.[20] Most of the active drug is eliminated unchanged in the urine and feces, with a minor fraction being further metabolized by conjugation to form pharmacologically active acyl glucuronides.[21]

Dabigatran metabolism does not seem to involve, inhibit, or induce CYP450 enzymes, which should minimize clinically relevant interactions with drugs metabolized by CYP450 and limit the effect of *CYP450* polymorphisms in drug response. Dabigatran does seem to be affected by polymorphisms in *CES1*. A GWAS in a subset of patients from the RE-LY study found that an SNP in this gene was associated with a decrease in dabigatran trough levels and reduced the risk of overall bleeding.[22] More than 30% of patients in RE-LY carried this SNP, and its effect was found to be greater than the effect of drug dosage.

Genetic determinants related to drug pharmacokinetics may also be relevant in dabigatran treatment. The prodrug dabigatran etexilate is a substrate for the p-glycoprotein drug efflux transporter encoded by the *ABCB1* gene.[23–25] The same GWAS from the subset of RE-LY patients found that the *ABCB*1 rs4148738 polymorphism is associated with an increase in peak plasma concentrations of dabigatran.[22] However, there was no association between dabigatran concentration and adverse events (ie, bleeding, ischemic events), making the clinical consequences of *ABCB1* polymorphisms on dabigatran bioavailability uncertain.

Factor Xa inhibitors—rivaroxaban, apixaban, edoxaban

Factor Xa inhibitors have been available clinically for only a short amount of time. Rivaroxaban was approved by the European Commission in 2008 and by US FDA in 2011 for deep vein thrombosis prophylaxis. Apixaban was approved for use in Europe in 2011 and in the United States in 2012, with its primary indication being risk reduction of stroke and systemic embolism in patients with nonvalvular atrial fibrillation. The most recent factor Xa inhibitor to be approved was edoxaban in 2015 in both the United States and Europe.

No literature exists to date on the clinical importance of pharmacogenetics in factor Xa therapeutics. However, each drug's known metabolic and pharmacokinetic profile suggests potential genetic determinants. All 3 drugs are directly pharmacologically active and reversibly inhibit factor Xa. In addition, all 3 drugs are substrates of CYP450, particularly CYP3A4/5 and CYP2J2, and of p-glycoprotein and, therefore, potentially influenced by *ABCB1* polymorphisms. One clinical trial aimed at determining the impact of genetic factors on dabigatran and rivaroxaban therapy has concluded, but results are not yet available,[26] and another trial examining the influence of *ABCB1* polymorphisms on plasma concentrations of dabigatran, rivaroxaban, and apixaban is ongoing.[27]

Nevertheless, results from studies comparing factor Xa inhibitors apixaban or edoxaban with warfarin therapy have demonstrated a safety benefit using the factor Xa inhibitor in some situations. The Apixaban for the Prevention of Stroke in Subjects With Atrial Fibrillation (ARISTOTLE) trial found apixaban was not only superior to warfarin in prevention of stroke and systemic embolism in patients with atrial fibrillation, but also was associated with fewer bleeding events and a reduction in mortality.[28] In the Global Study to Assess the Safety and Effectiveness of Edoxaban (DU-176b) vs Standard Practice of Dosing With Warfarin in Patients With Atrial Fibrillation (ENGAGE AF-TIMI) trial, *CYP2C9* and *VKORC1* variants were associated with bleeding events for patients taking warfarin but not edoxaban, providing evidence that edoxaban may be superior to warfarin for reducing the risk of bleeding in patients with these genotypes.[29]

ANTIPLATELET AGENTS

Platelets are central to the pathogenesis of atherothrombosis, stroke, and cardiovascular disease, which has led to both an increased interest in understanding platelet activation and aggregation, as well as the development of novel antiplatelet therapies.[30] Many oral antiplatelet agents, from the long-used aspirin to the newer P2Y12 antagonists clopidogrel, prasugrel, and ticagrelor, exhibit interindividual variability that may be influenced by genetics. Patients treated with P2Y12 inhibitors have variable degrees of platelet reactivity in laboratory-based assays, and such variability has clinical consequences. For example, studies have shown that patients treated with clopidogrel or prasugrel and have high residual platelet reactivity are at increased risk of ischemic events, whereas similarly treated patients with low platelet reactivity are at an increased risk of major bleeding.[31,32] The association of platelet reactivity with these severe clinical events underscores the importance of understanding how to achieve the optimal antiplatelet effect in each individual patient.

Acetylsalicylic Acid

Aspirin irreversibly acetylates the platelet enzyme prostaglandin G/H synthase-1 (cyclooxygenase-1), thereby decreasing thomboxane A2 generation from arachidonic acid and inhibiting platelet activation and ultimately thrombus formation.[33] Although the prevalence of "aspirin resistance" has garnered significant attention and controversy, it seems that platelet hyporesponsiveness to aspirin is often multifactorial and true nonresponse is rare.[34,35] Pharmacogenetic studies of aspirin responsiveness have investigated the impact of polymorphisms in various genes, including those encoding subunits of platelet receptors (ie, *ITGB3, ITGA2*) and those encoding the cyclooxygenases (ie, *PTGS1, PTGS2*), without clear evidence of the clinical impact of such genetic variations.[36] Nonresponse is often overcome clinically either by increasing the dose of aspirin or by adding a second antiplatelet agent, and current guidelines recommend dual treatment with aspirin and a P2Y12 inhibitor (ie, clopidogrel) for a synergistic effect in many clinical situations.[37]

P2Y12 Inhibitors

The platelet P2Y12 receptor is an adenosine diphosphate receptor that significantly mediates activation and aggregation, and P2Y12 receptor inhibitors have proven therapeutic value.[38,39] The P2Y12 antagonists include the irreversible thienopyridines, clopidogrel and prasugrel, and the reversible nonthienopyridine ticagrelor.

Thienopyridine P2Y12 inhibitors—clopidogrel and prasugrel

Clopidogrel was first approved for use in the United States in 1997 and became available in a generic formulation in 2012. It is primarily indicated for use in patients with acute coronary syndromes (ACS) or in patients with a recent history of ischemic stroke, MI, or established peripheral artery disease. Prasugrel was approved in the United States in 2009 for the reduction of thrombotic cardiovascular events in ACS patients undergoing percutaneous coronary intervention (PCI). Although both drugs demonstrate some degree of pharmacodynamic variability, prasugrel has greater bioavailability and is more potent than clopidogrel.[40–42] The P2Y12 Inhibitors Utilization in Bifurcation and Chronic Total Occlusion PCI (TRITON-TIMI 38) study, which compared treatment with prasugrel versus clopidogrel in patients with ACS undergoing PCI, found that prasugrel was associated with a significantly decreased risk of ischemic events but a significantly increased risk of major bleeding.[43]

Clopidogrel and prasugrel are both thienopyridine prodrugs that require activation by CYP450 enzymes to generate pharmacologically bioactive metabolites. Clopidogrel is converted predominantly to an inactive derivative, with only a minor fraction (~15%) undergoing the 2-sequential oxidation steps to generate the active metabolite.[44] CYP2C19, CYP3A4/5, and CYP1A2 enzymes are important in this bioactivation.[40]

Prasugrel metabolism is considered more efficient, with more than 50% of the drug becoming bioactivated, and primarily mediated by CYP3A4 and CYP2B6 enzymes.[40,45,46]

The effect of *CYP2C19* polymorphisms on clopidogrel therapy has been studied extensively. The *CYP2C19*2* loss-of-function allele was first reported in 2006 to be associated with decreased platelet responsiveness to clopidogrel.[47] Since then, numerous studies have confirmed this association, although it seems the *CYP2C19*2* genotype accounts for only a small fraction of variability in clopidogrel response.[48–50] A gain-of-function allele, *CYP2C19*17*, was found to be associated with increased biologic response to clopidogrel, but recent evidence suggests that this association depends on *CYP2C19*2* owing to linkage disequilibrium.[51]

The US FDA issued a label warning in 2009 and a boxed warning in 2010 alerting patients and health care professionals that clopidogrel treatment is less effective in patients with impaired CYP2C19 function (ie, patients who carry the *CYP2C19*2* allele). Currently, the Clinical Pharmacogenetics Implementation Consortium recommends that clinicians consider genotyping of *CYP2C19* in patients with ACS and undergoing PCI.[52]

Genetic polymorphisms in *CYP450* do not seem to influence prasugrel therapy significantly, although some studies do suggest an association.[53,54] Substudies on data available from TRITON-TIMI 38 did not find significant associations between common *CYP* variants and levels of active metabolites, platelet inhibition, or clinical cardiovascular event rates.[55,56] The authors noted a nonsignificant trend toward increased cardiovascular death, MI, or stroke in prasugrel-treated patients who carried the *CYP2B6* reduced-function allele, which warrants further study.[56]

Clopidogrel and prasugrel are both substrates of the p-glycoprotein efflux pump encoded by *ABCB1*. The clinical significance of *ABCB1* polymorphisms in clopidogrel pharmacodynamics is unclear. In 1 study, patients with the *ABCB1* C3435T genotype had decreased clopidogrel absorption and circulating metabolite plasma levels,[57] and in the TRITON-TIMI 38 study, this polymorphism was associated significantly with an increased risk of cardiovascular death, MI, or stroke in patients taking clopidogrel.[55] However, *ABCB1* was not a significant determinant of high platelet reactivity for patients taking clopidogrel in the GIFT study.[58] *ABCB1* genotype has not been a significant factor in pharmacologic or clinical outcomes in patients treated with prasugrel, a finding attributed to its rapid metabolism.[55]

Multiple studies have investigated the impact of still other genes on clopidogrel response variability. SNPs in other CYP450 enzymes relevant for clopidogrel metabolism, such as CYP2C9, CYP3A4, and CYP3A5, did not seem to affect clopidogrel response, nor did polymorphisms of paraoxonase-1 and P2Y12.[40] The GIFT study looked at 17 genes related to platelet reactivity in more than 1000 patients receiving standard or high-dose clopidogrel after PCI, and found the *CYP2C19*2* allele was the only significant genetic determinant associated with high on-treatment platelet reactivity.[58]

Nonthienopyridine P2Y12 inhibitor—ticagrelor

Ticagrelor is a P2Y12 inhibitor in the cyclopentyltriazolopyrimidine class that does not require bioactivation and instead acts directly and reversibly to exert an antiplatelet effect.[59] Metabolism occurs via CYP450, with CYP3A4 and CYP3A5 primarily responsible for the formation of the 2 major metabolites.[59,60]

Ticagrelor was approved for use in the United States in 2011 for the prevention of thrombotic events in patients with ACS or a history of MI. The A Comparison of Ticagrelor (AZD6140) and Clopidogrel in Patients With Acute Coronary Syndrome (PLATO) trial, which compared ticagrelor versus clopidogrel as treatment for patients with ACS, found that ticagrelor reduced the rate of death from vascular causes, MI, or stroke and was not associated with an increase in overall major bleeding, though there was an increase in the rate of non–procedure-related bleeding.[61]

Pharmacogenetic studies with ticagrelor are limited but have not found clinically significant associations between ticagrelor therapy and certain genotypes thus far. A small substudy from A Trial Comparing the Ischemic Preconditioning Effects of Ticagrelor and Clopidogrel in Humans (DISPERSE) and DISPERSE-2 trials assessed whether SNPs in *P2Y12, P2Y1,* or *ITGB3* influenced the pharmacodynamic response to ticagrelor in patients with stable atherosclerotic disease (DISPERSE) or ACS (DISPERSE-2), and found no association.[62] Data pooled from the Randomised, Double-Blind, Outpatient, Crossover Study of the Anti-platelet Effects of Ticagrelor Compared With Clopidogrel in Patients With Stable Coronary Artery Disease Previously Identified as Clopidogrel Non-responders or Responders (RESPOND) and Study of the Onset and Offset of Antiplatelet Effects Comparing Ticagrelor, Clopidogrel, and Placebo With Aspirin (ONSET/OFFSET) studies found no association between the antiplatelet effect of ticagrelor and *CYP2C19* or *ABCB1* genotypes.[63] Finally, data available from the PLATO trial were further investigated to search for potential genetic determinants, with at least 2 GWAS failing to find any significant effect of therapy-associated polymorphisms on clinical outcomes.[64,65] Taken together, the results of these studies suggest that individual drug responses to new antiplatelet agents prasugrel and ticagrelor are less affected by genetic polymorphisms than clopidogrel.

SUMMARY

Pharmacogenetics holds promise for preventing failures of antithrombotic therapy, both thrombosis from lack of efficacy and hemorrhage from excessive activity. Pharmacogenetic testing for *CYP2C9* and *VKORC1* polymorphisms can improve initial warfarin dosing, and testing for *CYP2C19* polymorphism can predict inadequate response to clopidogrel. Despite this, clinical use of genotype-tailored antithrombotic therapy is not widespread. This is in part owing to limited availability of laboratory testing and the cost associated with such strategies, but this may change as cost declines and if cost effectiveness can be shown.[66]

Another major reason for the limited adoption of pharmacogenetics is that genetic information, even when available, is regarded as 1 piece of data in a multifactorial clinical decision making process. A very recent prospective study looked at the propensity of cardiologists to choose antiplatelet therapy based on *CYP2C19* genotype as part of a pharmacogenetics implementation program.[67] Cardiologists were given the *CYP2C19* allele status for more than 90% of patients, and nearly 20% of patients in the study group (2676 stented patients) carried a *CYP2C19* variant affecting clopidogrel metabolism. Still, clinicians selected an alternative drug for only 57% of poor metabolizers and 33% of intermediate metabolizers. The authors concluded that, despite prescribers citing *CYP2C19* variant status as the most influential factor impacting drug selection, both genomic and nongenomic risks were important in clinical decision making.

Provider use of pharmacogenetic information will likely evolve as the ability to generate information about polymorphisms in single genes develops into an integrated understanding of variants in multiple gene networks. For example, despite the information pharmacogenetics has shown about clopidogrel and the *CYP2C19* loss of function allele, this variant is thought to account for only a small part (5%–12%) of the interindividual response.[36] Several studies show that high platelet reactivity in patients treated with clopidogrel seems to be only mildly influenced by nongenetic factors,[68–70] and some authors have suggested these known clinical factors account for about 10% of the drug variability.[36] As such, the majority of variability in clopidogrel response may be owing to as yet unidentified genetic causes.

Current studies are just beginning to provide the data necessary to realize the implementation of true "precision medicine" and these approaches will likely lead to changes in standard practice by incorporating pharmacogenetics into antithrombotic treatment decisions. Right now the use of pharmacogenetic information in anticoagulant and antiplatelet therapies seems to be limited and, in some cases, controversial. Still, given the continuing impact of genetic information in many aspects of health care, not to mention the recognition of the increasing financial burdens related to both venous and arterial vascular diseases, the need to incorporate genetic information as part of an improved, effective, personalized treatment plan for all vascular diseases will inevitably require knowledge of and use of pharmacogenetics.

Blood thinners have proven effects,

Optimum choices are hard to select.

To make therapy ample, genes must be sampled.

To identify drugs most correct.

REFERENCES

1. Valdes R, Al-Ghoul M. Fundamentals of pharmacology and applications in pharmacogenetics. Clin Lab Med 2008;28(4):485–97.
2. Weinshilboum R. Inheritance and drug response. N Engl J Med 2003;348: 529–37.
3. Pengo V, Pegoraro C, Cucchini U, et al. Worldwide management of oral anticoagulant therapy: the ISAM study. J Thromb Thrombolysis 2006;21:73–7.
4. Rettie AE, Korzekwa KR, Kunze KL, et al. Hydroxylation of warfarin by human cDNAexpressed cytochrome P450: a role for P4502C9 in the etiology of warfarin drug interactions. Chem Res Toxicol 1992;5(1):54–9.
5. Aithal GP, Day CP, Kesteven PJ, et al. Association of polymorphisms in the cytochrome P450 *CYP2C9* with warfarin dose requirement and risk of bleeding complications. Lancet 1999;353:717–9.
6. Furuya H, Fernandez-Salguero P, Gregory W, et al. Genetic polymorphism of CYP2C9 and its effect on warfarin maintenance dose requirement in patients undergoing anticoagulation therapy. Pharmacogenetics 1995;5:389–92.
7. Lindh JD, Holm L, Andersson ML, et al. Influence of CYP2C9 genotype on warfarin dose requirements- a systematic review and meta-analysis. Eur J Clin Pharmacol 2009;65:365–75.
8. Rost S, Fregin A, Ivaskevicius V, et al. Mutations in VKORC1 cause warfarin resistance and multiple coagulation factor deficiency type 2. Nature 2004;427:537–41.
9. Rieder MJ, Reiner AP, Gage BF, et al. Effect of VKORC1 haplotypes on transcriptional regulation and warfarin dose. N Engl J Med 2005;352:2285.
10. Cooper GM, Johnson JA, Langaee TY, et al. A genome-wide scan for common genetic variants with a large influence on warfarin maintenance dose. Blood 2008;112:1022–7.

11. Takeuchi F, McGinnis R, Bourgeois S, et al. A genome-wide association study confirms VKORC1, CYP2C9, and CYP4F2 as principle genetic determinants of warfrain dose. PLoS Genet 2009;5:e1000433.
12. Limdi NA, Brown TM, Yan Q, et al. Race influences warfarin dose changes associated with genetic factors. Blood 2015;126(4):539–45.
13. Klein TE, Altman RB, Eriksson N, et al. Estimation of the warfarin dose with clinical and pharmacogenomic data. N Engl J Med 2009;360:753–64.
14. Li X, Yang J, Wang X, et al. Clinical benefits of pharmacogenetic algorithm-based warfarin dosing: meta-analysis of randomized controlled trials. Thromb Res 2015; 135(4):621–9.
15. Ansell J, Hirsh J, Hylek E, et al. Pharmacology and management of the vitamin K anatagonists: American College of Chest Physicians Evidence-Based Clinical Practice Guidelines (8th Edition). Chest 2008;133:160S.
16. Fuster V, Bhatt DL, Califf RM, et al. Guided antithrombotic therapy: current status and future research direction. Circulation 2012;126:1645–62.
17. Shulman S, Kearon C, Kakkar AK, et al. Dabigatran versus warfarin in the treatment of acute venous thromboembolism. N Engl J Med 2009;361(24):2342–52.
18. Patel MR, Mahaffey KW, Garg J, et al. Rivaroxaban versus warfarin in nonvalvular atrial fibrillation. N Engl J Med 2001;365(10):883–91.
19. Eriksson BI, Smith H, Yasothan U, et al. Dabigatran etexilate. Nat Rev Drug Discov 2008;7(7):557–8.
20. Laizure SC, Parker RB, Herring VL, et al. Identification of carboxylesterase-dependent dabigatran etexilate hydrolysis. Drug Metab Dispos 2014;42(2): 201–6.
21. Blech S, Ebner T, Ludwig-Schwellinger E, et al. The metabolism and disposition of the oral direct thrombin inhibitor dabigatran in humans. Drug Metab Dispos 2008;36:386–99.
22. Pare G, Eriksson N, Lehr T, et al. Genetic determinants of dabigatran plasma levels and their relation to bleeding. Circulation 2013;127(13):1404–12.
23. Di Nisio M, Middeldorp S, Buller HR. Direct thrombin inhibitors. N Engl J Med 2005;353(10):1028–40.
24. Ishiguro N, Kishimoto W, Volz A, et al. Impact of endogenous esterace activity on in vitro p-glycoprotein profiling of dabigatran etexilate in Caco-2 monolayuers. Drug Metab Dispos 2014;42:250–6.
25. Hartter S, Koenen-Bergmann M, Sharma A, et al. Decrease in the oral bioavailability of dabigatran etexilate after co-medication with rifampicin. Br J Clin Pharmacol 2012;74:490–500.
26. New oral anticoagulant drugs dabigatran etexilate and rivaroxaban: influence of genetic factors in healthy volunteers. Available at: https://clinicaltrials.gov/ct2/show/NCT01627665. Accessed January 1, 2016.
27. Influence of ABCB1 polymorphisms on plasma concentrations of new oral anticoagulants in case of serious adverse events. Available at: https://clinicaltrials.gov/ct2/show/NCT02103101. Accessed January 1, 2016.
28. Granger CB, Alexander JH, McMurray JJV, et al. Apixaban versus warfarin in patients with atrial fibrillation. N Engl J Med 2011;365(11):981–92.
29. Mega JL, Walker JR, Ruff CT, et al. Genetics and the clinical response to warfarin and edoxaban: findings from the randomized double-blind ENGAGE AF-TIMI 48 trial. Lancet 2015;385(9984):2280–7.
30. Yousuf O, Bhatt DL. The evolution of antiplatelet therapy in cardiovascular disease. Nat Rev Cardiol 2011;8:547–59.

31. Tantry US, Bonello L, Aradi D, et al. Consensus and update on the definition of on-treatment platelet reactivity to adenosine diphosphate associated with ischemia and bleeding. J Am Coll Cardiol 2013;62:2261–73.

32. Aradi D, Kirtane A, Bonello L, et al. Bleeding and stent thrombosis on P2Y12-inhibitors: collaborative analysis on the role of platelet reactivity for risk stratification after percutaneous coronary intervention. Eur Heart J 2015;36(27):1762–71.

33. Undas A, Brummel-Ziedins KE, Mann KG. Antithrombotic properties of aspirin and resistance to aspirin: beyond strictly antiplatelet actions. Blood 2007; 109(6):2285–92.

34. Hankey GJ, Eikelboom JW. Aspirin resistance. Lancet 2006;367(9510):606–17.

35. Tantry US, Bliden KP, Gurbel PA. Overestimation of platelet aspirin resistance detection by thromboelastograph platelet mapping and validation by conventional aggregometry using arachidonic acid stimulation. J Am Coll Cardiol 2005;46(9):1705–9.

36. Storelli F, Youssef D, Desmeules J, et al. Pharmacogenomics of oral antithrombotic drugs. Curr Pharm Des 2016;22(13):1933–49.

37. Jneid H, Anderson JL, Wright RS, et al. 2012 ACCF/AHA focused update of the guideline for the management of patients with unstable angina/Non-ST-elevation myocardial infarction (updating the 2007 guideline and replacing the 2011focused update): a report of the American College of Cardiology Foundation/American Heart Association Task Force on practice guidelines. Circulation 2012;126(7):875–910.

38. Dorsam RT, Satya P, Kunapuli SP. Central role of the P2Y12 receptor in platelet activation. J Clin Invest 2004;113(3):340–5.

39. Yusuf S, Zhao F, Mehta SR, et al. Effects of clopidogrel in addition to aspirin in patients with acute coronary syndromes without ST-segment elevation. N Engl J Med 2001;345(7):494–502.

40. Ancrenaz V, Daali Y, Fontana P, et al. Impact of genetic polymorphisms and drug-drug interactions on clopidogrel and prasugrel response variability. Curr Drug Metab 2010;11(8):667–77.

41. Angiolillo DJ, Suryadevara S, Capranzano P, et al. Prasugrel: a novel platelet ADP P2Y12 receptor antagonist. A review on its mechanism of action and clinical development. Expert Opin Pharmacother 2008;9:2893–900.

42. Wallentin L, Varenhorst C, James S, et al. Prasugrel achieves greater and faster P2Y12 receptor-mediated platelet inhibition than clopidogrel due to more efficient generation of its active metabolite in aspirin-treated patients with coronary artery disease. Eur Heart J 2008;29:21–30.

43. Wiviott SD, Braunwald E, McCabe CH, et al. Prasugrel versus clopidogrel in patients with acute coronary syndromes. N Engl J Med 2007;357(20):2001–15.

44. Sangkuhl K, Klein ET, Altman RB. Clopidogrel pathway. Pharmacogenet Genomics 2010;20(7):463–5.

45. Rehmel JL, Eckstein JA, Farid NA, et al. Interaction of two major metabolites of prasugrel, a thienopyridine antiplatelet agent, with the cytochromes P450. Drug Metab Dispos 2006;34(4):600–7.

46. Payne CD, Li YG, Small DS, et al. Increased active metabolite formation explains the greater platelet inhibtion with prasugrel compared to high-dose clopidogrel. J Cardiovasc Pharmacol 2007;50(5):555–62.

47. Hulot JS, Bura A, Villard E, et al. Cytochrome P450 2C19 loss-of-function polymorphism is a major determinant of clopidogrel responsiveness in healthy subjects. Blood 2006;108(7):2244–7.

48. Shuldiner AR, O'Connell JR, Bliden KP, et al. Association of cytochrome P450 2C19 genotype with the antiplatelet effect and clinical efficacy of clopidogrel therapy. JAMA 2009;302(8):849–57.
49. Fontana P, James R, Barazer I, et al. Relationship between paraoxonase-1 activity, its Q192R genetic variant and clopidogrel responsiveness in the ADRIE study. J Thromb Haemost 2011;9(8):1664–6.
50. Hochholzer W, Trenk D, Fromm MF, et al. Impact of cytochrome P450 2C19 loss-of-function polymorphism and of major demographic characteristics on residual platelet function after loading and maintenance treatment with clopidogrel in patients undergoing elective coronary stent placement. J Am Coll Cardiol 2010; 55(22):2427–34.
51. Lewis JP, Stephens SH, Horenstein RB, et al. The CYP2C19*17 variant is not independently associated with clopidogrel response. J Thromb Haemost 2013;11(9): 1640–6.
52. Scott SA, Sangkuhl K, Stein CM, et al. Clinical Pharmacogenetics Implementation Consortium guidelines for CYP2C19 genotype and clopidogrel therapy: 2013 update. Clin Pharmacol Ther 2013;94:317–23.
53. Franken CC, Kaiser AF, Kruger JC, et al. Cytochrome P450 2B6 and 2C9 genotype polymorphism – a possible cause of prasugrel low responsiveness. Thromb Haemost 2013;110:131–40.
54. Cuisset T, Loosveld M, Morange PE, et al. CYP2C19*2 and *17 alleles have a significant impact on platelet response and bleeding risk in patients treated with prasugrel after acute coronary syndrome. JACC Cardiovasc Interv 2012;5:1280–7.
55. Mega JL, Close SL, Wiviott SD, et al. Genetic variants in ABCB1 and CYP2C19 and cardiovascular outcomes after treatment with clopidogrel and prasugrel in the TRITON-TIMI 38 trial: a pharmacogenetic analysis. Lancet 2010;376(9749): 1312–9.
56. Mega JL, Close SL, Wiviott SD, et al. Cytochrome P450 genetic polymorphisms and the response to prasugrel: relationship to pharmokinetic, pharmacodynamic, and clinical outcomes. Circulation 2009;119(19):2553–60.
57. Taubert D, von Beckerath N, Grimberg G, et al. Impact of p-glycoprotein on clopidogrel absorption. Clin Pharmacol Ther 2006;80(5):486–501.
58. Price MJ, Murray SS, Angiolillo DJ, et al. Influence of genetic polymorphisms on the effect of high and standard dose clopidogrel after percutaneous coronary intervention: the GIFT (Genotype Information and Functional Testing) study. J Am Coll Cardiol 2012;59(22):1928–37.
59. Teng R. Ticagrelor: pharmacokinetic, pharmacodynamic, and pharmacogenetic profile: an update. Clin Pharmacokinet 2015;54(11):1125–38.
60. Teng R, Oliver S, Hayes MA, et al. Absorption, distribution, metabolism, and excretion of ticagrelor in healthy subjects. Drug Metab Dispos 2010;38(9): 1514–21.
61. Wallentin L, Becker RC, Budaj A, et al. Ticagrelor versus clopidogrel in patients with acute coronary syndromes. N Engl J Med 2009;361:1045–57.
62. Storey RF, Melissa Thornton S, Lawrance R, et al. Ticagrelor yields consistent dose-dependent inhibition of ADP-induced platelet aggregation ni patients with atherosclerotic disease regardless of genotypic variations in P2RY12, P2RY1, and ITGB3. Platelets 2009;20:341–8.
63. Tantry US, Bliden KP, Wei C, et al. First analysis of the relation between CYP2C19 genotype and pharmacodynamics in patients treated with ticagrelor versus clopidogrel: the ONSET/OFFSET and RESPOND genotype studies. Circ Cardiovasc Genet 2010;3(6):556–66.

64. Akerblom A, Eriksson N, Wallentin L, et al. Polymorphism of the cystatin C gene in patients with acute coronary syndromes: results from the Platelet Inhibition and Patient Outcomes Study. Am Heart J 2014;168:96–102.e2.

65. Varenhorst CMH, Eriksson N, Johansson Å, et al. Ticagrelor plasma levels but not clinical outcomes are associated with transporter and metabolism enzyme genetic polymorphisms. J Am Coll Cardiol 2014;63(12_S):A25.

66. Sweezy T, Mousa SA. Genotype-guided use of oral antithrombotic therapy: a pharmacoeconomic perspective. Personalized Medicine 2014;11(2):223–35.

67. Peterson J, Field J, Unertl K, et al. Physician response to implementation of genotype-tailored antiplatelet therapy. Clinical Pharmacology & Therapeutics 2016. [Epub ahead of print].

68. Fontana P, Berdague P, Castelli C, et al. Clinical predictors of dual aspirin and clopidogrel poor responsiveness in stable cardiovascular patients from the ADRIE study. J Thromb Haemost 2010;8:2614–23.

69. Gremmel T, Steiner S, Seidinger D, et al. Adenosine disphosphate-inducible platelet reactivity shows a pronounced age dependency in the initial phase of antiplatelet therapy with clopidogrel. J Thromb Haemost 2010;8:37–42.

70. Tidjane MA, Voisin S, Lhermusier T, et al. More on: adenosine disphosphate-inducible platelet reactivity shows a pronounced age dependency in the initial phase of antiplatelet therapy with clopidogrel. J Thromb Haemost 2011;9:614–6.

Laboratory Medicine in the Clinical Decision Support for Treatment of Hypercholesterolemia

Pharmacogenetics of Statins

Gualberto Ruaño, MD, PhD[a],*, Richard Seip, PhD[b],
Andreas Windemuth, PhD[c], Alan H.B. Wu, PhD[d],
Paul D. Thompson, MD[e]

KEYWORDS

- Statins • Myopathy • Coenzyme Q_{10} • Pharmacogenetics • Physiogenomics
- Myalgia • Lipid metabolism • PCSK9 inhibitors

KEY POINTS

- Genotype–phenotype associations in large cohorts have confirmed loci at APOB, APOE-APOC1-APOC4-APOC2, LDLR, HMGCR, and proprotein convertase subtilisin/kexin 9 (PCSK9) that are associated with low-density lipoprotein cholesterol (LDLC) in patients with elevated cholesterol.
- Variants in the gene that encodes cholesteryl ester transport protein, though not associated with total LDLC, have been linked to LDLC subfractions.
- Research has linked polymorphisms in the SLCO1B1 gene to elevated serum creatine kinase activity (myalgia) in patients receiving simvastatin therapy.

Continued

Supported in part by the NIGMS NIH Small Business Innovation Research Grant R44 GM-085201 *System for DNA-Guided Optimization and Personalization of Statin Therapy*. The ClinicalTrials. gov identifier for the SINM study is NCT00767130. Dr G. Ruaño is Principal Investigator of the study and President and Founder of Genomas Inc. The views presented in this article are strictly those of the authors, and do not represent the opinions of the companies Genomas Inc, Sanofi, or Cyclica that employ, respectively, Dr G. Ruaño, Dr R. Seip, and Dr A. Windemuth. Dr A.B.H. Wu and Dr P.D. Thompson report no conflicts.

[a] Genomas Inc., 67 Jefferson Street, Hartford, CT 06106, USA; [b] Sanofi Genzyme, 500 Kendall Street, Cambridge, MA 02142, USA; [c] Cyclica Inc., 10 Jonathan Street, Belmont, MA 02478, USA; [d] Department of Laboratory Medicine, San Francisco General Hosptial, 1001 Potrero Avenue, San Francisco, CA 94110, USA; [e] Division of Cardiology, Hartford Hospital, 80 Seymour Street, Hartford, CT 06106, USA
* Corresponding author.
E-mail address: g.ruano@genomas.net

Clin Lab Med 36 (2016) 473–491
http://dx.doi.org/10.1016/j.cll.2016.05.010
0272-2712/16/$ – see front matter © 2016 Elsevier Inc. All rights reserved.

labmed.theclinics.com

Continued

- COQ2, ATP2B1, and DMPK, representing pathways involved in myocellular energy transfer, calcium homeostasis, and myotonic dystonia, respectively, have been validated as markers for the common myalgia observed in patients receiving statin therapy, and integrated into a physiogenomic predictive model for myalgia diagnosis and prognosis in clinical therapeutics.
- Statin pharmacogenetics is expected to play a significant role in the selection and confirmation of patients for PCSK9 inhibitors.

PERSONALIZED MEDICINE OF STATINS

One of the promises of the Human Genome Project is individualization of patient care based on highly heterogeneous innate metabolic factors determined by DNA typing of gene polymorphisms. Translation of such gene polymorphisms into clinical decision support for personalized health care is the basis for DNA-guided medicine. Statin responsiveness is an area of high research interest given the success of the drug class in the treatment of hypercholesterolemia, and in primary and secondary prevention of cardiovascular disease (CVD). Interrogation of the patient's genetic status for variants will eventually guide hyperlipidemic intervention.

Statins selectively and competitively inhibit the intracellular enzyme hydroxymethylglutaryl coenzyme A (HMGCoA) reductase that is expressed to different degrees in various tissues. HMGCoA reductase is the rate-limiting enzyme in cholesterol biosynthesis.

In addition to the inhibition of cholesterol synthesis, the inhibition of HMGCoA activity reduces synthesis of geranyl and farnesyl products, leading to decreased isoprenylation of proteins and possible impairment of many varied cellular functions. Statin entry into cells can be gated, and metabolic pathways for the drugs of this class are varied and drug-dependent.

Statins are the most prescribed drugs in the United States[1] and the world.[2] Atorvastatin, simvastatin, and rosuvastatin make up 85% of the prescriptions written in the United States.[1] The success of this drug class in primary and secondary prevention of CVD[3] has fostered increasingly aggressive use and dosing.

STATIN EFFICACY

Administered at maximum dosages, the most common statins (ie, atorvastatin, simvastatin, rosuvastatin, and pravastatin) lower low-density lipoprotein (LDL) cholesterol (LDLC) by 37% to 57% in patients with primary hypercholesterolemia.[4–7] The magnitude of the LDLC response differs according to phenotypic, demographic, and as yet unexplained characteristics.[8]

Although approximately 50% of the variability in plasma LDLC is estimated to be due to inheritance,[9] only a small number of common and multiple rare gene variants that contribute to the phenotype are known.[9–11] Pharmacogenetic studies of LDLC-lowering associated with statin therapy have focused mainly on genes in cholesterol synthetic, lipoprotein lipid transport, and pharmacokinetic pathways, showing that single nucleotide polymorphisms (SNPs) in genes of cholesterol metabolism, such as *HMGCR*,[12–15] and lipoprotein transport, such as *APOE*[15–24] and *LIPC*,[25] can influence the statins' ability to lower LDLC levels. Variants in pharmacokinetic genes, such as *SLCO1B1* that encodes the organic ion transporter protein 1B1, and *CYP7A1* that encodes the cytochrome p450 7A1 protein, can also affect LDLC-lowering with statins.[24,26] Recent findings have begun to extend the repertoire of gene variants associated with statin efficacy to new mechanisms of drug action. The *KIF6* gene codes for a cytoskeletal protein involved in intracellular transport of protein complexes, membrane organelles, and messenger RNA (mRNA).[27] The Trp719Arg substitution in the protein enhances the efficacy of statin therapy, apparently through pleiotropic effects.[28] In the absence of statin therapy, variants in genes, such as *APOE*,[29–31] *APOB*,[30,31] *NPC1L1*,[32] *PSCK9*,[31,33] *CELSR2*,[30] *PSRC1*,[30] *SORT1*,[30,31] and *LDLR*,[9,30,31] affect LDLC. Because baseline LDLC predicts, to some extent, the magnitude of LDLC-lowering with statins, there may be overlap in the genes that regulate LDLC metabolism and statin-mediated LDLC-lowering.

The authors' previous physiogenomic studies have generated hypothetical mechanisms related to statin-induced myositis[34] and myalgia.[35] The authors have also used physiogenomic analysis to further investigate gene associations to LDLC in subjects receiving statin therapy.[36] The authors found new evidence of opposing effects associated with an intronic variant near the ACACB mitochondrial-binding domain, rs34274, and an SNP near the cyclic adenosine monophosphate (cAMP)-dependent phosphorylation site, rs2241220, to LDLC-lowering in subjects receiving statin therapy (**Fig. 1**). This study used a cohort of 202 subjects receiving statin therapy and genotyped for an array consisting of 384 SNPs distributed across physiologic pathways represented by 222 genes.

Genotype–phenotype associations in large cohorts have confirmed loci at *APOB*, *APOE-APOC1-APOC4-APOC2*, *LDLR*, *HMGCR*, and *PCSK9*,[10] and discovered intergenic SNPs in the chromosomal regions 1p13 (near *CELSR2*, *PSRC1*, and *SORT1*) and 19p13 (near *CILP2* and *PBX4*)[10] that are associated with LDLC in subjects with elevated cholesterol. Genome-wide studies have shown that common, noncoding SNPs in HMGCoA reductase are significantly associated with LDLC levels but that the effect sizes are relatively small, a 5% difference in LDL level.[10] The addition of

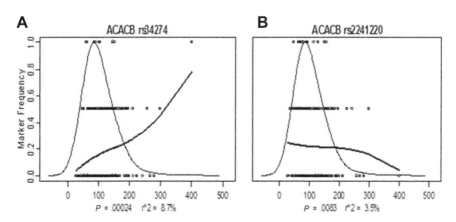

Fig. 1. Associations with LDLC lowering through *ACACB* rs34274 (*A, left*) and *ACACB* rs2241220 (*B, right*). Each circle represents a subject (genotype), with the horizontal axis specifying the LDLC, and the vertical axis the genotype. Bottom circles, homozygous for major allele; middle circles, heterozygous; top circles, homozygous for minor allele. A locally-weighted scatter plot smoothing (LOESS) fit of the allele frequency as a function of LDLC (*thick line*) is shown. (*From* Ruaño G, Thompson PD, Kane JP, et al. Physiogenomic analysis of statin-treated patients: domain-specific counter effects within the ACACB gene on low-density lipoprotein cholesterol? Pharmacogenomics. 2010;11(7):965; with permission.)

genotype scoring, consisting of summing the number of risk markers among the 11 SNPs just mentioned, has significantly improved risk classification in CVD-prone subjects in large cohorts.

In addition, variants in the gene that encodes cholesteryl ester transport protein (CETP), though not associated with total LDLC, have been linked to LDL subfractions.[37] LDL subfractions vary in atherogenicity, and variability in activity of the cholesteryl ester transport protein is hypothesized to play a role the modification of their size and density. In this regard, the investigation of CETP haplotypes in relation to LDL subfractions warrants further investigation.[38]

STATIN SAFETY

The main clinically relevant safety risk is statin-induced neuromyopathy evidenced as a constellation of neuromuscular side effects. Neuromyopathies are disabling to 3% to 20% of patients on statins, require alteration of therapy, and reduce compliance.[35,39–41] Neuromyopathies include myalgias (pain, weakness, aches, cramps) and myositis (typically monitored by elevation of serum creatine kinase [CK] activity).[39] Neuromyopathies vary in extent among drugs and from patient to patient. Were there a system to predict the safety and efficacy of the pre-eminent statin drugs according to the genome of each patient, a clinician could optimize the selection from among atorvastatin, simvastatin, and rosuvastatin. Alternatively, a patient's genomic profile may prove incompatible with statins and the clinician could decide to avoid the drug class.

The authors have considered myalgias and myositis independently under the broader diagnosis of myopathy. Often, myalgias occur in patients with no or little CK elevation and CK is not necessarily elevated in the presence of histopathological evidence of statin-associated muscle damage.[36,42] Only in the clinically rare condition of rhabdomyolysis is the relationship between myopathy, extremely elevated CK, and clinical severity incontrovertible.[43] There is a need to identify novel surrogate markers that can better predict high risk of myalgia in patients taking statins.[12]

Despite the limitations of CK measurement with respect to its specificity to statin neuromyopathy,[44] in clinical studies, increased activity of serum CK has provided the predominant means for assessing the degree of myopathic severity. The elevation of CK activity to 10-fold upper limit of normal indicates severe statin-induced neuromyopathy.[45] Pharmacokinetic gene-focused hypotheses are based on the increased plasma statin concentrations resulting from decreased first-pass hepatic clearance (variation in drug transporters) and metabolism (variation in cytochrome p450 and glucuronidation pathways).[46]

Previous research linked polymorphisms in the *SLCO1B1* gene to elevated serum CK activity (myalgia) in subjects receiving simvastatin therapy. *SLCO1B1* encodes for the OATB1 protein (organic anion transporter B1), which is a regulator of hepatic statin uptake. In patients selected for a high degree of CK elevation, the pharmacokinetic gene *SLCO1B1* *5 variant rs4363657 SNP is associated with CK elevation,[42] likely through linkage disequilibrium with the nonsynonymous SNP rs4149056 (Val174Ala) or the rs4149080 SNP in the 13th intron.[47] The relationship between *SLCO1B1* and CK elevation has been independently confirmed.[47] This association may be simvastatin-specific and not an effect seen with all statins.

A subsequent report assessed *SLCO1B1* polymorphisms in relation to clinically reported myalgia during rosuvastatin therapy.[48] Subjects enrolled in the Justification for the Use of Statins in Prevention: an Intervention Trial Evaluating Rosuvastatin (JUPITER) trial without prior CVD or diabetes who had LDLC less than 130 mg/dL and C-reactive protein greater than or equal to 2 mg/L were randomly allocated to rosuvastatin 20 mg or placebo and followed for first CVD events and adverse effects. The SNPs rs4363657 and rs4149056 in *SLCO1B1* were assessed for association with clinically reported myalgia, which was determined as self-reported symptoms. Clinical myalgia frequency over 1.9 years of follow-up was not different between rosuvastatin and placebo, and the investigators conclude that myalgia is not associated with the SNPs of interest in subjects taking rosuvastatin.

Phenotypic expression of myalgia is quite variable[40,49] and mechanistic explanations of the pharmacodynamic bases of neuromuscular side effects have incorporated diverse and complex pathways.[39,41] These have been recently summarized.[50] Statin interactions with HMGCoA reductase homologue proteins may interfere with energy transduction processes.[51,52] Some mechanisms find their basis in the possibility that statin inhibition of nonsteroidal molecules, such as ubiquinone and isoprenoid, triggers disruption in normal mitochondrial function, cell signaling, cell proliferation, and cell repair.[39,51,53–62] Specific proposed myalgia causes include decreased sarcolemmal[39] or sarcoplasmic reticular cholesterol,[63] reduced production of ubiquinone or coenzyme Q_{10},[64] decreased prenylated proteins,[39,65] changes in fat metabolism,[66] increased uptake of cholesterol[67] or phytosterols,[68] failure to replace damaged muscle protein via the ubiquitin pathway,[69] disruption of calcium metabolism in the skeletal muscle,[70,71] and inhibition of selenoprotein synthesis.[56] Pharmacodynamic genetic markers are generally unknown, though progress to identify candidate markers has been made.[50] Vladutiu[72] reported increased prevalence of heterozygosity among known markers for several inherited muscle metabolic diseases.

Two approaches are illustrated: hypothesis-free genome-wide association studies and hypothesis-led candidate gene studies.

Hypothesis-Free Approach: Genome-Wide Single Nucleotide Polymorphism Associations

The authors pursued a hypothesis-free genome-wide association study (GWAS) probing the association of 865,483 SNPs across all chromosomes in a group of 812 outpatients undergoing statin therapy for hyperlipidemia.[73] The study sample was enriched with subjects diagnosed as having statin-induced neuromyopathy, accomplished through recruitment of subjects treated at specialized lipid clinics. The results confirmed the association of 3 out of 31 previously identified candidate genes, including *COQ2* and *CPT2*, involved in myocellular energy transfer and provided a novel association through the neuronally expressed *CLN8* gene. The Manhattan plot in **Fig. 2** shows the association of log-scores for all 865,483 SNPs to myalgia as a

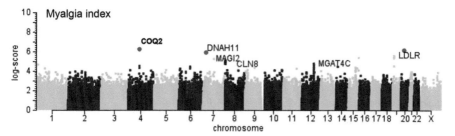

Fig. 2. Manhattan plot for myalgia index. The scale on the ordinate represents statistical significance as the log-score ($s = -\log_{10} p$) and the abscissa represents the chromosomal location, with the chromosome boundaries indicated by the coloring of the data points. The strongest SNP associations (log-score >5) are indicated by a filled circle (●), and the top 6 markers are labeled with the name of the associated gene for 865,483 SNPs.

function of their genomic location. In GWAS, the Manhattan plot is a scatter diagram in which genomic location coordinates are displayed along the X-axis, whereas the negative logarithm of the associated statistical probability (P)-value for each SNP is displayed on the Y-axis. Thus each dot on the Manhattan plot signifies an SNP. The strongest associations have the greatest height because the negative logarithms of the smallest P-values will be the greatest values. For example, a P-value of 10^{-10} will have a value of 10 in the plot.

At a threshold log-score of 7.2 (calculated from the negative logarithm$_{10}$ of 0.05 ÷ 865,483), no associations reached genome-wide significance after correction for the 865,483 multiple comparisons. However, there are several interesting associations that are suggestive. The full set of suggestive associations is listed in **Table 1**. The highest log-score in the study, 6.3, was achieved by SNP rs4693570 on chromosome 4, located 100 kb downstream of the gene for para-hydroxybenzoate polyprenyltransferase (COQ2), whose enzyme product catalyzes a final reactions in the biosynthesis of coenzyme Q$_{10}$. COQ2 was also one of the top candidate genes. SNP rs11980747, with a log-score of 6.1 ($P<2\cdot10^{-6}$, correlation coefficient [R^2] = 3.1%), is located within the gene for the heavy chain of axonemal dynein (DNAH11). SNPs rs2738466, rs14158, rs2116897, and rs2569537 on chromosome 19 were associated with log-scores of 5.6, 5.5, 5.4, and 5.3, respectively ($P<5\cdot10^{-6}$, R^2 = 2.9%), and located in linkage within the gene for low-density lipoprotein receptor (LDLR). At a log-score of 5.1 ($P<10^{-5}$, R^2 = 2.6%), there is SNP rs7014327, located within the gene ceroid-lipofuscinosis, neuronal 8 (CLN8).

Fig. 3 shows the genomic locus and the SNP effect on myalgia for the 4 genes identified previously. The figures show log-scores of association for all SNPs within 200 kilobase (kb) of the index SNP along the chromosome and, on the right, show the effect of the variant allele on the probability of myalgia in subgroups of subjects taking 1 of the 3 major statins. In all cases, the loci show linkage disequilibrium, indicated because there are other associated SNPs in the direct vicinity of the index SNP. Interestingly, the CLN8 SNP shows a very strong drug-dependent effect. There is no effect at all in the group of subjects taking either rosuvastatin or simvastatin but a strong effect ($P<2\cdot10^{-7}$, R^2 = 5.2%) in the group of subjects taking atorvastatin. The difference in effect between the subpopulations is significant ($P<.05$) under the t-statistic.

Not shown but also interesting at P less than 10^{-5}, corresponding to a log-score of 5.0 or better, are 2 additional SNPs not associated with any gene and an SNP in the gene MAGI2, membrane-associated guanylate kinase, WW, and PDZ domain. The protein encoded by MAGI2 interacts with atrophin-1. Atrophin-1 contains a polyglutamine repeat, the expansion of which is responsible for dentatorubral and pallidoluysian atrophy. This encoded protein is characterized by 2 WW domains, a guanylate kinase-like domain, and multiple PDZ domains. It has structural similarity to the membrane-associated guanylate kinase homologue (MAGUK) family. The threshold ($P<10^{-5}$) represents a posterior likelihood of true association of greater than 10%. SNP rs7267722, on chromosome 20 with a log-score of 6.1 ($P<7\cdot10^{-7}$, R^2 = 3.3%), is not associated with any gene and located in the middle of an approximately 400 kb intergenic region.

Hypothesis-Led Approach: Validation of Candidate Genes

The authors also assembled a list of 31 candidate genes with known or hypothetical pharmacodynamic or pathologic roles in myalgia assessed from several previous publications. **Table 2** lists the candidates with literature references and the authors' validation results. There are 9 genes with an adjusted log-score higher than 1.3 ($P<.05$) and 3 that are statistically significant in the face of multiple comparisons among loci: COQ2 ($P<3\cdot10^{-5}$), ATP2B1 ($P<.001$), and DMPK ($P<.002$).

e associations for myalgia index at a suggestive significance level ($P<10^{-5}$)

Chromosome	Log-Score	Coefficient	Frequency	Correlation Coefficient	Symbol	Gene Name
4	6.3	0.11	58%	3.3%	COQ2	Coenzyme Q10 (100 kb downstream)
7	6.1	−0.25	95%	3.2%	DNAH11	Dynein, axonemal, heavy chain 11
20	6.1	0.09	36%	3.3%	rs7267722	No gene link
9	5.6	−0.12	26%	2.9%	LDLR	LDL receptor
9	5.5	0.12	73%	2.9%	LDLR	LDL receptor
5	5.5	−0.10	36%	2.9%	rs1023781	No gene link
9	5.4	0.12	73%	2.8%	LDLR	LDL receptor
7	5.3	−0.12	76%	2.8%	MAGI2	Membrane-associated guanylate kinase, WW domain containing 2
9	5.3	0.12	73%	2.8%	LDLR	LDL receptor
8	5.1	−0.10	31%	2.6%	CLN8	Ceroid-lipofuscinosis, neuronal 8 (epilepsy, p with mental retardation)

he negative logarithm of the P-value. A log-score of 5 corresponds to P-value of 10^{-5}.

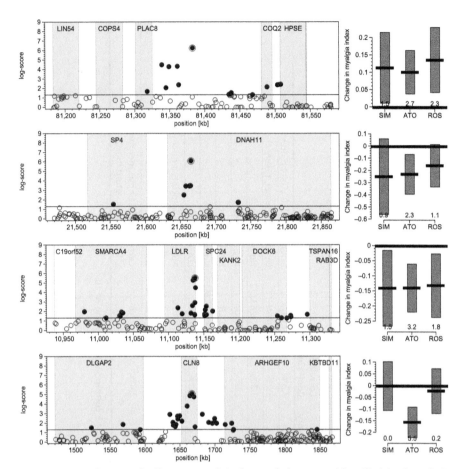

Fig. 3. Genomic locus and effect on myalgia for 4 of the genes identified in the whole-genome screen. The panels show log-scores of association for all SNPs within 200 kb of the index SNP along the chromosome and, on the right, show the effect of the variant allele on the probability of myalgia in subgroups of patients taking 1 of the 3 major statins. ([*Top panel*] *From* Ruaño G, Windemuth A, Wu AH, et al. Mechanisms of statin-induced myalgia assessed by physiogenomic associations. Atherosclerosis 2011;218(2):454; with permission.)

COQ2

The *COQ2* gene encodes mitochondrial para-hydroxybenzoate-polyprenyltransferase, an enzyme that catalyzes 1 of the final reactions in the biosynthesis of coenzyme $Q10_{10}$ (CoQ_{10}), the prenylation of para-hydroxybenzoate with an all-trans poly-prenyl group.[74] CoQ_{10} (ubiquinone) serves as a redox carrier in the mitochondrial respiratory chain and is a lipid-soluble antioxidant. CoQ_{10} blood concentrations are lowered by statins, and CoQ_{10} deficiency has been linked to mitochondrial myopathy.

DMPK

The *DMPK* gene encodes myotonin-protein kinase (*MT-PK*), a serine-threonine kinase that has been implicated in myotonic dystrophy type I, an inherited multi-systemic disease characterized by wasting of the muscles (muscular dystrophy), cataracts, heart conduction defects, endocrine changes, and myotonia. Newly diagnosed patients with inherited myopathies have been reported to have a higher exposure rate to statins,[75] suggesting that statins may have contributed to the onset of symptoms.

CLN8

The authors identified a new candidate, *CLN8*, which has a strong effect only in patients taking atorvastatin and not taking either rosuvastatin or simvastatin. *CLN8* has not been implicated directly with myopathy but it is associated with Pompe disease, which in turn has been associated with statin-induced myopathy. Its drug-dependent association supports the hypothesis that the myopathy side effect is mediated by different pathways for different statins. Further research to elucidate the biological association of *CLN8* with myopathy and statins, and to confirm its association in a follow-up study of subjects treated with statins is needed.

Compared with other recent GWAS studies, this study is limited in statistical power but it is the largest examination of statin-induced myalgia to date. The associations determined in the authors' study confirm connections between common myalgia and genes involved in biochemical pathways that have been previously implicated in statin myalgia. Other candidate genes tested here were not validated. One of these, the *SLCO1B1* gene demonstrates variants that are strongly associated with elevated CK during simvastatin therapy.[42,47] The authors' study[73] observed a different phenotype and tested only a limited number of subjects receiving simvastatin. The present study detected no association of *SLCO1B1* to myalgia, probably as a consequence of its broader set of statins and phenotype.

The authors successfully validated *COQ2*, *ATP2B1*, and *DMPK* as candidate genes for statin-induced myalgia. The candidate genes, *COQ2*, *ATP2B1*, and *DMPK*, representing pathways involved in myocellular energy transfer, calcium homeostasis, and myotonic dystonia, respectively, were validated as markers for the common myalgia observed in subjects receiving statin therapy.

MULTIGENE MODELS

These 3 genes integrated into a physiogenomic predictive model could be relevant to myalgia diagnosis and prognosis in clinical therapeutics. The authors had identified a clear tendency for the risk alleles (*COQ2*-G, *DMPK*-G, and *ATP2B1*-T) to be dominant, and there was a substantial effect of each allele on the probability of developing myalgia.[73] The genotypic effect of the markers on the probability of myalgia is detailed in **Fig. 4**. The combined effect of the 3 markers is quantified, showing that of the 2 subjects with no risk alleles, none have myalgia, and of the 40 subjects with the full complement of 6 risk alleles, 70% have myalgia. The study confirmed 3 previously identified markers. Among the 377 subjects diagnosed clinically as having statin myalgia, all have at least 1 risk allele from the 3 validated genes.

The Statin Induction and Neuro-Myopathy (SINM) study sought to identify genetic markers for statin myopathy that can be used to predict which subjects are most likely to develop myopathic complaints during statin treatment and to aid in objectifying the diagnosis of statin myopathy. Combining the *COQ2*, *ATP2B1*, and *DMPK* markers into a physiogenomic panel to represent candidate pathways and deriving a risk score, establishes a prototype system to predict the onset of myalgia and to aid in diagnosis.[73] Despite subjectivity in diagnosis of statin myalgia, the study identified previously suspected candidate genes with logical relationships to muscle metabolism as contributing to statin myalgia.

es and their associations to myalgia index

hologic Finding	Chromosome	Symbol	Log-Score	Gene
ptors[35]	11	HTR3B	ns	5-Hydroxytryptamine (serotonin) receptor 3B
	10	HTR7	ns	5-Hydroxytryptamine (serotonin) receptor 7
transporter[42]	12	SLCO1B1	ns	Solute carrier organic anion transporter family, m
34	3	AGTR1	ns	Angiotensin II receptor, type 1
	7	NOS3	1.4	Nitric oxide synthase 3 (endothelial cell)
	17	ACE	ns	Angiotensin I converting enzyme (peptidyl-dipept
orylase[41]	11	PYGM	2.0	Phosphorylase, glycogen, muscle
	17	GAA	ns	Glucosidase, alpha; acid
ed[41]	11	CPT1A	ns	Carnitine palmitoyltransferase 1A (liver)
	22	CPT1B	ns	Carnitine palmitoyltransferase 1B (muscle)
	1	CPT2	ns	Carnitine palmitoyltransferase II
deaminase[41]	1	AMPD1	ns	Adenosine monophosphate deaminase 1 (isoform
energy[41]	4	COQ2	4.4	Coenzyme Q2 homolog, prenyltransferase (yeast)
	9	APTX	ns	Aprataxin
ophy[40]	19	DMPK	2.8	Dystrophia myotonica-protein kinase
	X	DMD	ns	Dystrophin
	18	AQP4	ns	Aquaporin 4

ort[41]	12	**ATP2B1**	**3.1**	**ATPase, Ca++ transporting, plasma membrane 1**
	16	ATP2A1	ns	ATPase, Ca++ transporting, cardiac muscle, fast t
	17	ATP2A3	ns	ATPase, Ca++ transporting, ubiquitous
	19	RYR1	ns	Ryanodine receptor 1 (skeletal)
	1	RYR2	ns	Ryanodine receptor 2 (cardiac)
	3	ATP2B2	1.5	ATPase, Ca++ transporting, plasma membrane 2
	3	ATP2C1	1.5	ATPase, Ca++ transporting, type 2C, member 1
	7	RYR3	1.7	Ryanodine receptor 3
	X	ATP2B3	ns	ATPase, Ca++ transporting, plasma membrane 3
	16	ATP2C2	ns	ATPase, Ca++ transporting, type 2C, member 2
	12	ATP2A2	ns	ATPase, Ca++ transporting, cardiac muscle, slow
	1	ATP2B4	1.8	ATPase, Ca++ transporting, plasma membrane 4
otubule dynamics[41]	8	FAM82B	ns	Family with sequence similarity 82, member B
e disease[41]	3	CAV3	ns	Caveolin 3

he negative algorithm of the association *P*-value for each gene. Log-scores greater than 1.3 (*P*<.05) are shown. Log-scores 2.8 or gre atistically significant (bold font) after adjusting for testing of 31 multiple genes in the selected set of candidates (Bonferroni corr t shown and are reported as ns (not significant).

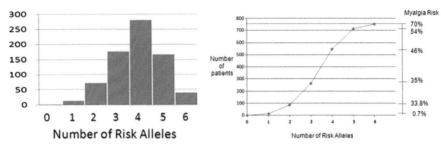

Fig. 4. (*Left*) Frequency distribution showing the numbers of patients carrying from 0 to 6 risk alleles, respectively, at the 3 polymorphic sites rs4693570 (*COQ2*, para-hydroxybenzoate-polyprenyltransferase), rs6732348 (*DMPK*, myotonin, protein kinase), and rs17381194 (plasma membrane calcium-transporting ATPase 1). All patients were treated with statins and approximately 40% were diagnosed with statin myalgia. (*Right*) Statin myalgia risk index curve based on the same SNP markers. According to the function, a patient with 0 or 1 risk allele has less than 1% chance of experiencing myalgia on statin. A patient with 5 risk alleles has a 54% chance and a patient with 6 risk alleles, a 70% chance. As the number of predictive SNP markers in the model is increased, it may be possible to refine further the prediction of statin myalgia beyond 70%.

BIOTECHNOLOGY DRUGS FOR TREATMENT OF HYPERCHOLESTEROLEMIA

Over the last 5 years, the pharmaceutical industry has developed new therapies, such as nucleic acid antisense compounds and monoclonal antibodies, for the treatment of severe genetic hypercholesterolemia. These molecules may be extended to treatment of patients who are refractory or intolerant of statin treatment.

One such mRNA inhibitor is mipomersen, an antisense oligonucleotide that specifically binds to *APOB* mRNA, rendering it susceptible to degradation. Mipomersen inhibits hepatic formation and release of nascent apolipoprotein B100-containing lipoproteins and can lower LDLC in patients whose LDL particle recognition and hepatic uptake mechanism is defective. Another drug, lomitapide, a small molecule inhibitor of microsomal triglyceride transfer protein, inhibits transfer of lipid into developing chylomicrons in enterocytes and very LDL particles in hepatocytes, resulting in fewer apolipoprotein B100- and B48-containing particles. At present these agents remain specifically targeted to patients with confirmed genetic homozygous hypercholesterolemia.

Monoclonal antibodies have been synthesized to inhibit proprotein convertase subtilisin/kexin 9 (PCSK9) activity. Through binding to PCSK9, the inhibitors disrupt the intracellular traffic that normally degrades the LDL receptor. PCSK9 antibodies seem effective and safe in phase III trials. In the class, 2 monoclonal antibodies produced by different pharmaceutical companies were approved by the Food and Drug Administration as of late 2015. The agents are indicated for use in patients with heterozygous familial cholesterolemia and/or patients with atherosclerotic vascular disease on maximally tolerated statins, who require additional LDL reduction. The US target population for these drugs, when patients who are unable to tolerate maximal statin therapy are included, is sizable. In the Understanding Statin Use in America and Gaps in Patient Education (USAGE) study, a survey of approximately 10,000 current and former statin users, 12% of subjects on statins discontinued therapy and 62% of these subjects cited side effects as the reason for discontinuation.[76] More than 86% of subjects who discontinued therapy because of side effects cited muscle pain or weakness as the reason. Based on these data, it has been estimated that approximately 6% of statin users, representing more than 2 million adults in the United States, ceased therapy because of muscle pain or weakness and are, therefore, statin intolerant.[77] The authors expect statin pharmacogenetics to play a significant role in the selection and confirmation of patients unlikely to be well managed with the more conventional and far less expensive statins.

Clinical Scenarios

Statins will remain the first-line therapy in the foreseeable future for patients with high CVD risk that is traditionally founded on elevated LDLC. The authors have created a prototype decision-support matrix that incorporates statin-specific SNP markers of both efficacy and safety with the intent to provide decision-making guidance. The quantitative comparison of the merits of each drug offers more clinical resolution than generalized single-drug outcomes.[78] With such pharmacogenetic decision-support tools, the value to the physician is the capacity to address the complexity and variety of clinical scenarios and appropriately evaluate the need for nonstatin drugs. **Fig. 5** describes 3 clinical scenarios from actual records of patients in the authors' clinical registry.

Scenario 1

The patient was a white man with history of statin therapy for elevated cholesterol and a successful reduction in LDLC to a level of 85 mg/dL with statin therapy, well below the target level of 100 mg/dL. Statin-associated myopathy was diagnosed by the treating physician. Analysis of the patient's genome, focused on genotypes of the decision-support matrix, did not reveal a statin-wide adversity but clear and dramatic differences in predicted safety and efficacy among the 3 statins.

#1 Drug / Phenotype	Myalgia Index	logCK	LDL
Rosuvastatin	0.51 (77%)	5.38 (81%)	256.75 (97%)
Atorvastatin	0.22 (47%)	4.48 (40%)	137.15 (65%)
Simvastatin	0.28 (54%)	-2.24 (0%)	42.57 (2%)

#2 Drug / Phenotype	Myalgia Index	logCK	LDL
Rosuvastatin	0.02 (26%)	5.00 (67%)	162.89 (81%)
Atorvastatin	-0.70 (0%)	4.24 (27%)	115.87 (51%)
Simvastatin	0.04 (28%)	0.93 (0%)	207.37 (93%)

#3 Drug / Phenotype	Myalgia Index	logCK	LDL
Rosuvastatin	-0.13 (14%)	5.76 (90%)	78.66 (23%)
Atorvastatin	-0.16 (13%)	5.46 (84%)	175.25 (86%)
Simvastatin	-0.04 (21%)	-1.64 (0%)	209.41 (93%)

Fig. 5. SINM PhyzioType results and drug recommendations for 3 patients (#1, #2, #3). The PhyzioType Result is a matrix defined by predictions for 3 phenotypes (Myalgia Index, locCK, LDL) in response to 3 drugs (rosuvastatin, atorvastatin, simvastatin). The values on the left of the cells are predicted responses, with percentile ranks in parentheses on the right. The color coding of the cells with the predictions for each patient represents their quartile rank in a population distribution: Red, worst quartile with unfavorable response; green, best quartile with favorable response; yellow, second and third quartiles with intermediate response.

According to the decision-support matrix, simvastatin is preferred based on predicted responses in the lowest quartiles for predicted log CK (low CK activity) and predicted LDLC (42 mg/dL) (green cells), and predicted responses for myalgia that were in the middle 2 quartiles of patient distributions. In contrast, the SINM PhyzioType predicts undesirable responses for all 4 parameters (myalgia, plasma CK activity, LDLC, high-density lipoprotein cholesterol) for rosuvastatin (red cells) and safety and efficacy responses to atorvastatin that are not highly favorable or unfavorable (yellow cells). This patient would not be a candidate for PCSK9 inhibitor.

Scenario 2

This patient had been previously treated with simvastatin 5 mg, atorvastatin 10 mg, and rosuvastatin 10 mg. The patient complained of mild discomfort on each of the drugs but the physician was unconvinced and diagnosed possible statin-associated myopathy. The LDLC level was 189 mg/dL. In this case, the decision-support matrix provided a clinical guidance toward atorvastatin as the best choice of statin to treat the patient's hypercholesterolemia based on predicted LDLC level of 115.9 mg/dL, which is an efficacy prediction that is favorable compared with rosuvastatin and simvastatin but still subpar. The support matrix is already pointing to limitations of statin treatment, which may cause this patient to be treated with statin as a last trial in anticipation of a switch to PCSK9 inhibitor.

Scenario 3

The patient had been treated with lovastatin 20 mg, which lowered LDLC to 88 mg/dL (satisfying target goal achievement) but caused mild discomfort that was interpreted by the treating clinician as possible statin-associated myalgia. Rosuvastatin 5 mg was subsequently tried. In this case, the decision-support matrix revealed no clear superior statin for treatment. Rosuvastatin had the best profile based on highly favorable efficacy with respect to predicted LDLC level of 78.7 mg/dL and the prediction of low myalgia risk but of an elevated CK (ln[CK] = 5.76, or 317 CK activity units) presents a major risk. This patient would be a good candidate for PCSK9 inhibitors.

CLINICAL PHARMACOGENETIC TESTING

Testing for cardiovascular risk factors is available from direct-to-consumer companies. Selected clinical laboratories specializing in high-resolution lipid profiling have begun offering heart disease markers as an adjunct service.

Several academic centers and commercial laboratories have embraced *SLCO1B1* testing and have begun offering it clinically. However, this marker is limited to extreme myopathy, and seems to be simvastatin-specific. Commercial insurers in the United States do not cover the test.

Testing for myopathies is available from the Robert Guthrie Biochemical and Molecular Genetics Laboratory at SUNY Buffalo.[72] It is implemented for genetic myopathies but not for statin-related effects.

In June 2011, Genomas Inc announced a product development grant from the National Institute of General Medical Sciences to develop genetic tests and DNA-guided diagnostic systems for optimal selection of statins and for improved delivery of statin therapy for the treatment of CVD, obesity, and diabetes. This pioneering project is in progress and harbors the potential to provide clinicians and physicians with newly developed genetic tests and a decision-support system that will allow them to manage statins, prescribe and dose these drugs on a DNA-guided, personalized basis to more effectively guide the therapy for each patient. This decision support may be relevant to the prescription of biotechnology drugs to statin intolerant and recalcitrant patients.

Genetic testing for statin efficacy and safety is thus currently available but faces questions about its clinical utility and validity by the health care payers. The authors predict, however, that such testing will become standard once its economic value and return on the investment is demonstrated in selected instances.

REFERENCES

1. Findlay S. Prescription and price trends October 2005 to December 2006 and potential cost savings to Medicare from increased use of lower cost statins. Consumer Reports. 2-19-2007. Yonkers, NY, Consumers Union., in Consumer Reports. Yonkers (NY): Consumers Union; 2007.
2. Visiongain L. Statins: the world market, 2009-2024. London: 2009.
3. Waters DD. What the statin trials have taught us. Am J Cardiol 2006;98(1):129–34.
4. Jones P, Kafonek S, Laurora I, et al. Comparative dose efficacy study of atorvastatin versus simvastatin, pravastatin, lovastatin, and fluvastatin in patients with hypercholesterolemia (the CURVES study). Am J Cardiol 1998;81(5):582–7.
5. Stein EA, Davidson MH, Dobs AS, et al. Efficacy and safety of simvastatin 80 mg/day in hypercholesterolemic patients. The Expanded Dose Simvastatin U.S. Study Group. Am J Cardiol 1998;82(3):311–6.
6. Ballantyne CM, Weiss R, Moccetti T, et al. Efficacy and safety of rosuvastatin 40 mg alone or in combination with ezetimibe in patients at high risk of cardiovascular disease (results from the EXPLORER study). Am J Cardiol 2007;99(5):673–80.
7. Sacks FM, Moyé LA, Davis BR, et al. Relationship between plasma LDL concentrations during treatment with pravastatin and recurrent coronary events in the Cholesterol and Recurrent Events trial. Circulation 1998;97(15):1446–52.
8. Simon JA, Lin F, Hulley SB, et al. Phenotypic predictors of response to simvastatin therapy among African-Americans and Caucasians: the Cholesterol and Pharmacogenetics (CAP) Study. Am J Cardiol 2006;97(6):843–50.
9. Burnett JR, Hooper AJ. Common and rare gene variants affecting plasma LDL cholesterol. Clin Biochem Rev 2008;29(1):11–26.
10. Kathiresan S, Melander O, Guiducci C, et al. Six new loci associated with blood low-density lipoprotein cholesterol, high-density lipoprotein cholesterol or triglycerides in humans. Nat Genet 2008;40(2):189–97.
11. Kathiresan S, Melander O, Anevski D, et al. Polymorphisms associated with cholesterol and risk of cardiovascular events. N Engl J Med 2008;358(12):1240–9.
12. Chasman DI, Posada D, Subrahmanyan L, et al. Pharmacogenetic study of statin therapy and cholesterol reduction. JAMA 2004;291(23):2821–7.
13. Krauss RM, Mangravite LM, Smith JD, et al. Variation in the 3-hydroxyl-3-methylglutaryl coenzyme a reductase gene is associated with racial differences in low-density lipoprotein cholesterol response to simvastatin treatment. Circulation 2008;117(12):1537–44.
14. Polisecki E, Muallem H, Maeda N, et al. Genetic variation at the LDL receptor and HMG-CoA reductase gene loci, lipid levels, statin response, and cardiovascular disease incidence in PROSPER. Atherosclerosis 2008;200(1):109–14.
15. Thompson JF, Hyde CL, Wood LS, et al. Comprehensive whole-genome and candidate gene analysis for response to statin therapy in the Treating to New Targets (TNT) cohort. Circ Cardiovasc Genet 2009;2(2):173–81.
16. Donnelly LA, Palmer CN, Whitley AL, et al. Apolipoprotein E genotypes are associated with lipid-lowering responses to statin treatment in diabetes: a Go-DARTS study. Pharmacogenet Genomics 2008;18(4):279–87.

17. Maitland-van der Zee AH, Jukema JW, Zwinderman AH, et al. Apolipoprotein-E polymorphism and response to pravastatin in men with coronary artery disease (REGRESS). Acta Cardiol 2006;61(3):327–31.

18. Tavintharan S, Lim SC, Chan YH, et al. Apolipoprotein E genotype affects the response to lipid-lowering therapy in Chinese patients with type 2 diabetes mellitus. Diabetes Obes Metab 2007;9(1):81–6.

19. Pedro-Botet J, Schaefer EJ, Bakker-Arkema RG, et al. Apolipoprotein E genotype affects plasma lipid response to atorvastatin in a gender specific manner. Atherosclerosis 2001;158(1):183–93.

20. Sousa MO, Corbella E, Alía P, et al. Lack of association between the APOE genotype and the response to statin treatment in patients with acute ischemic episodes. Med Clin (Barc) 2008;130(11):401–4 [in Spanish].

21. Pena R, Lahoz C, Mostaza JM, et al. Effect of apoE genotype on the hypolipidaemic response to pravastatin in an outpatient setting. J Intern Med 2002;251(6):518–25.

22. Chiodini BD, Franzosi MG, Barlera S, et al. Apolipoprotein E polymorphisms influence effect of pravastatin on survival after myocardial infarction in a Mediterranean population: the GISSI-Prevenzione study. Eur Heart J 2007;28(16):1977–83.

23. Thompson JF, Man M, Johnson KJ, et al. An association study of 43 SNPs in 16 candidate genes with atorvastatin response. Pharmacogenomics J 2005;5(6):352–8.

24. Zhang W, Chen BL, Ozdemir V, et al. SLCO1B1 521T–>C functional genetic polymorphism and lipid-lowering efficacy of multiple-dose pravastatin in Chinese coronary heart disease patients. Br J Clin Pharmacol 2007;64(3):346–52.

25. Zambon A, Deeb SS, Brown BG, et al. Common hepatic lipase gene promoter variant determines clinical response to intensive lipid-lowering treatment. Circulation 2001;103(6):792–8.

26. Takane H, Miyata M, Burioka N, et al. Pharmacogenetic determinants of variability in lipid-lowering response to pravastatin therapy. J Hum Genet 2006;51(9):822–6.

27. Hirokawa N, Noda Y. Intracellular transport and kinesin superfamily proteins, KIFs: structure, function, and dynamics. Physiol Rev 2008;88(3):1089–118.

28. Iakoubova OA, Sabatine MS, Rowland CM, et al. Polymorphism in KIF6 gene and benefit from statins after acute coronary syndromes: results from the PROVE IT-TIMI 22 study. J Am Coll Cardiol 2008;51(4):449–55.

29. Bennet AM, Di Angelantonio E, Ye Z, et al. Association of apolipoprotein E genotypes with lipid levels and coronary risk. JAMA 2007;298(11):1300–11.

30. Chasman DI, Paré G, Zee RY, et al. Genetic loci associated with plasma concentration of low-density lipoprotein cholesterol, high-density lipoprotein cholesterol, triglycerides, apolipoprotein A1, and Apolipoprotein B among 6382 white women in genome-wide analysis with replication. Circ Cardiovasc Genet 2008;1(1):21–30.

31. Willer CJ, Sanna S, Jackson AU, et al. Newly identified loci that influence lipid concentrations and risk of coronary artery disease. Nat Genet 2008;40(2):161–9.

32. Cohen JC, Pertsemlidis A, Fahmi S, et al. Multiple rare variants in NPC1L1 associated with reduced sterol absorption and plasma low-density lipoprotein levels. Proc Natl Acad Sci U S A 2006;103(6):1810–5.

33. Cohen JC, Boerwinkle E, Mosley TH Jr, et al. Sequence variations in PCSK9, low LDL, and protection against coronary heart disease. N Engl J Med 2006;354(12):1264–72.

34. Ruaño G, Thompson PD, Windemuth A, et al. Physiogenomic analysis links serum creatine kinase activities during statin therapy to vascular smooth muscle homeostasis. Pharmacogenomics 2005;6(8):865–72.

35. Ruaño G, Thompson PD, Windemuth A, et al. Physiogenomic association of statin-related myalgia to serotonin receptors. Muscle Nerve 2007;36(3):329–35.

36. Ruaño G, Thompson PD, Kane JP, et al. Physiogenomic analysis of statin-treated patients: domain-specific counter effects within the ACACB gene on low-density lipoprotein cholesterol? Pharmacogenomics 2010;11(7):959–71.

37. Shim H, Chasman DI, Smith JD, et al. A multivariate genome-wide association analysis of 10 LDL subfractions, and their response to statin treatment, in 1868 Caucasians. PLoS One 2015;10(4):e0120758.

38. Winkelmann BR, Hoffmann MM, Nauck M, et al. Haplotypes of the cholesteryl ester transfer protein gene predict lipid-modifying response to statin therapy. Pharmacogenomics J 2003;3(5):284–96.

39. Thompson PD, Clarkson P, Karas RH. Statin-associated myopathy. JAMA 2003; 289(13):1681–90.

40. Bruckert E, Hayem G, Dejager S, et al. Mild to moderate muscular symptoms with high-dosage statin therapy in hyperlipidemic patients–the PRIMO study. Cardiovasc Drugs Ther 2005;19(6):403–14.

41. Ghatak A, Faheem O, Thompson PD. The genetics of statin-induced myopathy. Atherosclerosis 2010;210(2):337–43.

42. SEARCH Collaborative Group, Link E, Parish S, Armitage J, et al. SLCO1B1 variants and statin-induced myopathy–a genomewide study. N Engl J Med 2008; 359(8):789–99.

43. Ruaño G, Windemuth A, Holford TR. Physiogenomics: integrating systems engineering and nanotechnology for personalized medicine. In: Bronzino JD, editor. The biomedical engineering handbook. Cleveland (OH): CRC Press; 2005. p. 1–9.

44. Seip RL, Rivera N, Ruaño G, et al. Statin-induced neuromyopathy. In: Murray MF, Babyatsky MW, Giovanni MA, editors. Clinical genomics. Practical applications in adult care. New York: McGraw-Hill Education; 2014. p. 38–44.

45. McKenney JM, Davidson MH, Jacobson TA, et al. Final conclusions and recommendations of the National Lipid Association Statin Safety Assessment Task Force. Am J Cardiol 2006;97(8A):89C–94C.

46. Seip RL, Duconge J, Ruaño G. Genotype-guided statin therapy. In: Wu AHB, Yeo J, editors. Pharmacogenomic testing in current clinical practice: implementation in the clinical laboratory. New York: Humana Press, Springer Science+Business Media; 2011. p. 155–74.

47. Voora D, Shah SH, Spasojevic I, et al. The SLCO1B1*5 genetic variant is associated with statin-induced side effects. J Am Coll Cardiol 2009;54(17):1609–16.

48. Danik JS, Chasman DI, MacFadyen JG, et al. Lack of association between SLCO1B1 polymorphisms and clinical myalgia following rosuvastatin therapy. Am Heart J 2013;165(6):1008–14.

49. Stroes ES, Thompson PD, Corsini A, et al. Statin-associated muscle symptoms: impact on statin therapy-European Atherosclerosis Society Consensus panel Statement on assessment, aetiology and management. Eur Heart J 2015; 36(17):1012–22.

50. Needham M, Mastaglia FL. Statin myotoxicity: a review of genetic susceptibility factors. Neuromuscul Disord 2014;24(1):4–15.

51. Rosenson RS. Current overview of statin-induced myopathy. Am J Med 2004; 116(6):408–16.

52. Wilke RA, Mareedu RK, Moore JH. The pathway less traveled: moving from candidate genes to candidate pathways in the analysis of genome-wide data from large scale pharmacogenetic association studies. Curr Pharmacogenomics Person Med 2008;6(3):150–9.

53. Arora R, Liebo M, Maldonado F. Statin-induced myopathy: the two faces of Janus. J Cardiovasc Pharmacol Ther 2006;11(2):105–12.

54. Law M, Rudnicka AR. Statin safety: a systematic review. Am J Cardiol 2006; 97(8A):52C–60C.

55. Phillips PS, Haas RH, Bannykh S, et al. Statin-associated myopathy with normal creatine kinase levels. Ann Intern Med 2002;137(7):581–5.

56. Moosmann B, Behl C. Selenoprotein synthesis and side-effects of statins. Lancet 2004;363(9412):892–4.

57. Sinzinger H, Schmid P, O'Grady J. Two different types of exercise-induced muscle pain without myopathy and CK-elevation during HMG-Co-enzyme-A-reductase inhibitor treatment. Atherosclerosis 1999;143(2):459–60.

58. Franc S, Dejager S, Bruckert E, et al. A comprehensive description of muscle symptoms associated with lipid-lowering drugs. Cardiovasc Drugs Ther 2003; 17(5–6):459–65.

59. Sewright KA, Clarkson PM, Thompson PD. Statin myopathy: incidence, risk factors, and pathophysiology. Curr Atheroscler Rep 2007;9(5):389–96.

60. Dirks AJ, Jones KM. Statin-induced apoptosis and skeletal myopathy. Am J Physiol Cell Physiol 2006;291(6):C1208–12.

61. Hanai J, Cao P, Tanksale P, et al. The muscle-specific ubiquitin ligase atrogin-1/MAFbx mediates statin-induced muscle toxicity. J Clin Invest 2007;117(12): 3940–51.

62. Hansen KE, Hildebrand JP, Ferguson EE, et al. Outcomes in 45 patients with statin-associated myopathy. Arch Intern Med 2005;165(22):2671–6.

63. Draeger A, Monastyrskaya K, Mohaupt M, et al. Statin therapy induces ultrastructural damage in skeletal muscle in patients without myalgia. J Pathol 2006;210(1): 94–102.

64. Marcoff L, Thompson PD. The role of coenzyme Q10 in statin-associated myopathy: a systematic review. J Am Coll Cardiol 2007;49(23):2231–7.

65. Santos RD. What are we able to achieve today for our patients with homozygous familial hypercholesterolaemia, and what are the unmet needs? Atheroscler Suppl 2014;15(2):19–25.

66. Phillips PS, Haas RH. Statin myopathy as a metabolic muscle disease. Expert Rev Cardiovasc Ther 2008;6(7):971–8.

67. Yokoyama M, Seo T, Park T, et al. Effects of lipoprotein lipase and statins on cholesterol uptake into heart and skeletal muscle. J Lipid Res 2007;48(3):646–55.

68. Paiva H, Thelen KM, Van Coster R, et al. High-dose statins and skeletal muscle metabolism in humans: a randomized, controlled trial. Clin Pharmacol Ther 2005;78(1):60–8.

69. Urso ML, Clarkson PM, Hittel D, et al. Changes in ubiquitin proteasome pathway gene expression in skeletal muscle with exercise and statins. Arterioscler Thromb Vasc Biol 2005;25(12):2560–6.

70. Mohaupt MG, Karas RH, Babiychuk EB, et al. Association between statin-associated myopathy and skeletal muscle damage. CMAJ 2009;181(1–2):E11–8.

71. Guis S, Figarella-Branger D, Mattei JP, et al. In vivo and in vitro characterization of skeletal muscle metabolism in patients with statin-induced adverse effects. Arthritis Rheum 2006;55(4):551–7.

72. Vladutiu GD. Genetic predisposition to statin myopathy. Curr Opin Rheumatol 2008;20(6):648–55.
73. Ruaño G, Windemuth A, Wu AH, et al. Mechanisms of statin-induced myalgia assessed by physiogenomic associations. Atherosclerosis 2011;218(2):451–6.
74. Forsgren M, Attersand A, Lake S, et al. Isolation and functional expression of human COQ2, a gene encoding a polyprenyl transferase involved in the synthesis of CoQ. Biochem J 2004;382(Pt 2):519–26.
75. Sailler L, Pereira C, Bagheri A, et al. Increased exposure to statins in patients developing chronic muscle diseases: a 2-year retrospective study. Ann Rheum Dis 2008;67(5):614–9.
76. Cohen JD, Brinton EA, Ito MK, et al. Understanding Statin Use in America and Gaps in Patient Education (USAGE): an internet-based survey of 10,138 current and former statin users. J Clin Lipidol 2012;6(3):208–15.
77. Esperion Therapeutics Inc. Targeting Unmet Patient Needs: Finding new therapies for lowering LDLC for patients with hypercholesterolemia and a history of statin intolerance and for patients with residual risk. Plymouth (MI): 2013. p. 1–5. Available at: http://www.esperion.com/wp-content/uploads/2013/06/Esperion-Target-Needs-Whitepaper.pdf. Accessed May 22, 2016.
78. Ridker PM, Danielson E, Fonseca FA, et al. Rosuvastatin to prevent vascular events in men and women with elevated C-reactive protein. N Engl J Med 2008;359(21):2195–207.

Pharmacogenetics and Personalized Medicine in Pain Management

Lynn R. Webster, MD[a],*, Inna Belfer, MD, PhD[b,c]

KEYWORDS

- Pharmacogenetics • Polymorphism • Cytochrome P450 (CYP) • Genomic testing
- Pain management

KEY POINTS

- Individual genetic imprint affects pain perception and response to analgesics; environmental factors influence how this genetic profile is expressed.
- Recent research indicates multiple gene-gene and gene x environment interactions that influence pain and analgesia as well as common pathways among painful diseases.
- Studies of genetic polymorphisms linked to pain syndromes and medication metabolism herald a fresh therapeutic approach based on genotype with targeted analgesia and fewer side effects.
- Genome-wide association studies are needed to identify full genetic signatures for pain and analgesia and to underpin genetic testing in clinical practice.

INTRODUCTION

Pharmacogenetic therapy in pain patients requires consideration of 2 different genetic substrates to determine the outcome of pharmacotherapy. The first is the genetic contribution to a variety of different pain types, and the second is the genetic influence on drug effectiveness and safety. This article presents evidence of a genetic influence on the prevalence and processing of pain, a discussion of the genetics of drug treatment, and a clinical scenario to illustrate the need to integrate the genetics of pain and pharmacogenetics to achieve the best outcomes.

Financial Disclosures: L.R. Webster has received consulting, advisory board, and/or travel fees from AstraZeneca, Cara Therapeutics, Depomed, Egalet, INSYS Therapeutics, Jazz Pharmaceuticals, Kaleo Therapeutics, Marathon Pharmaceuticals, Merck, Orexo Pharmaceuticals, Pfizer, Proove Biosciences, Shionogi, Trevena, and Zogenix. I. Belfer has no financial disclosures.
[a] Scientific Affairs, PRA Health Sciences, 3838 South 700 East, Suite 202, Salt Lake City, UT 84106, USA; [b] Department of Medicine, University of Pittsburgh, 3550 Terrace Street, Pittsburgh, PA 15261, USA; [c] Department of Human Genetics, University of Pittsburgh, Pittsburgh, PA, USA
* Corresponding author.
E-mail address: lrwebstermd@gmail.com

GENETICS OF PAIN

Studies to isolate the genetic risk of inheriting a specific pain condition are plentiful, but scientists are only beginning to examine genetic variations that may influence pain processing. If a genetic basis underlies how pain is expressed and perceived, including the varying mechanisms of nociceptive, neuropathic, and visceral pain, then the potential exists for new analgesic targets affecting these gene products. In the future, the right drug may depend on the patient's genotype; furthermore, the genetic signature of personal analgesic response may guide both drug and drug dose selection. Pain expression is also influenced by environmental factors, such as cultural attitudes, attention, sleep, and stress. Fibromyalgia (FM), tension headaches, and irritable bowel syndrome are a few of the functional pain conditions influenced by environmental factors. It is increasingly recognized that complex phenotypes encompass genetic and environmental interactions that may shape predisposition to pain processing and perception.[1]

Candidate Gene Studies in Pain

Clinical observation of patients suggests large interindividual differences in pain sensitivity (**Fig. 1**), and research confirms that view.[2] Examples of pain conditions that persist in a minority of patients include diabetes with diabetic peripheral neuropathy, herpes zoster with postherpetic neuralgia, lumbar disc degeneration with low back pain, and whiplash injuries with cervicalgia.[3] Age, sex, severity of stimulus, and environmental factors explain some of the variance, but not all. A genetic influence is suggested by results showing that inbred mouse strains respond differently to the same acute and chronic pain stimuli.[4–6] Similarly, studies of sensitivity to painful stimulation showed a great variability in both threshold and tolerance to mechanical, thermal, and chemical stimuli in normal volunteers, only a tiny portion of which is explained by personality or expectations.[2]

Allele-based association studies have been expected to shed light on why pain persists in some patients but not in others after nearly identical tissue damage. Close to 200 candidate genes that may be involved in pain processing have been categorized by their frequency of occurrence in chronic neuropathic pain conditions and by the strength of evidence, frequency of the specific variant, and likelihood that a genetic polymorphism alters function. A polymorphism is a variation in DNA sequencing that occurs in greater than 1% of the population; in contrast, a mutation occurs in less than 1%[7] (**Table 1**).[3,8]

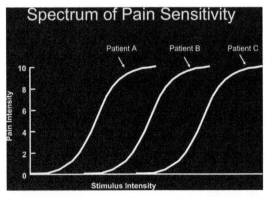

Fig. 1. A simulation of interindividual variability in pain sensitivity: patient A has increased sensitivity; patient B has a normal response, and patient C has decreased sensitivity.

Table 1
High-priority candidate genes for human neuropathic pain

Gene	Molecule	Single-Nucleotide Polymorphisms	Location
IL6	Interleukin-6	G 174 C	Promoter
NOS1	Neuronal nitric oxide synthase	AAT VNTR	Intron 20
IL1B	Interleukin-1β	C 511 T	Promoter
TNF α	Tumor necrosis factor-α	G 308 A	Promoter
SLC6A4	Serotonin transporter	5HTTLPR	Promoter
GDNF	Glial-derived nerve factor	(AGG) (n)	3′ Untranslated region
BDKRB2	Bradykinin receptor 2	C 58 T	Promoter
COMT	Catechol-O-methyltransferase	Val 158 Met	Exon 3
NOS2A	Inducible nitric oxide synthase	CCTTTn repeat	Promoter
PDYN	Prodynorphin	68-bp repeat	Promoter
OPRM1	μ-Opioid receptor	Asn 40 Asp	Exon 1
IL10	Interleukin-10	A 1082 G	Promoter
BDKRB1	Bradykinin receptor 1	G 699 T	Promoter
TH	Tyrosine hydroxylase	Val 81 Met	Exon 3
RET	Proto-oncogene (tyrosine kinase)	Gly 691 Ser	Exon 11
GRIK3	Kainate (glutamate) receptor	Ser 310 Ala	Coding
IL13	Interleukin-13	Arg 130 Gln	Coding
BDNF	Brain-derived nerve factor	Val 66 Met	Exon 5
ADRA2A	α₂ₐ-Adrenergic receptor	C 1291 G	Promoter
CACNA2D2	Calcium channel subunit	G 845 C	Intron 2

Promoter = a region of DNA that initiates transcription of a particular gene. Exon = a segment of a DNA or RNA molecule containing information coding for a protein or peptide sequence. Intron = a segment of a DNA or RNA molecule that does not code for proteins and interrupts the sequence of genes.

Data from Belfer I, Wu T, Kingman A, et al. Candidate gene studies of human pain mechanisms: methods for optimizing choice of polymorphisms and sample size. Anesthesiology 2004;100(6):1562–72; and Gilbert SC. Developmental biology. 6th edition. Sunderland (MA): Sinauer Associates; 2000. Available at: http://www.ncbi.nlm.nih.gov/books/NBK10023/. Accessed February 15, 2016.

More recent genetic and genomic technologies have allowed a genome-wide association unbiased study approach to complex pain traits. These studies revealed an underlying multilevel genetic architecture of pain control with many loci of different effect sizes, gene-gene interactions, and common pathways among painful diseases.[9] **Table 2** lists some of the studies showing genes that have been associated with pain processing and perception.[10] **Table 3** reports on genes found to reduce pain or be protective from pain.[11–18] **Table 4** elucidates some findings regarding the association of genetic variants with specific pain conditions and opioid dependence.[19–24]

Separating genetic from environmental factors is usually best explored through twin studies. In a study using classic twin design, a consistent excess concordance in monozygotic compared with dizygotic twins equated to up to 68% heritability for low back pain and up to 58% for neck pain.[25,26] The following subsections further elucidate findings related to genetics in specific pain conditions.

Table 2
Genes involved in the pain genome

Type	Example
Cytokones	*IL6, IL10, TNF*
Enzymes	*COMT, GCH1, CYP2D6*
Ion channels	*KCNS1, CACNG2, CACNA2D3*
Receptors	*OPRM1, ADRA2, DRD2*
Transporters	*DAT1, 5HTT, ABCB1*

From Belfer I. Personalized pain medicine: pharmacogenetic testing for pain and opioid addiction. Pain Medicine News 2015. Available at: http://www.painmedicinenews.com/Review-Articles/Article/09-15/Personalized-Pain-Medicine-Pharmacogenetic-Testing-for-Pain-and-Opioid-Addiction/33480/ses=ogst. Accessed February 22, 2016; with permission.

Table 3
Genes that reduce or protect from pain

Gene	Encoding
COMT	Catechol-O-methyltransferase
GCH1	Guanosine triphosphate cyclohydrolase 1
MC1R	Melanocortin-1 receptor
OPRM1	μ-Opioid receptor
TRPV1	Transient receptor potential cation channel

Data from Refs.[11–18]; and *From* Belfer I. Personalized pain medicine: pharmacogenetic testing for pain and opioid addiction. Pain Medicine News 2015. Available at: http://www.painmedicinenews.com/Review-Articles/Article/09-15/Personalized-Pain-Medicine-Pharmacogenetic-Testing-for-Pain-and-Opioid-Addiction/33480/ses=ogst. Accessed February 22, 2016; with permission.

Table 4
Genetic variants attributed to pain conditions, opioid use

Genetic Variant	Association
A region on chromosome 5p15.2, located upstream of chaperonin-containing TCP1-complex-5 gene and downstream of *FAM173B*	Associated with a 30% higher risk for chronic widespread pain
Common variants within the *ALDH1A2* gene and with rare variants at 1p31	Associated with severe osteoarthritis
Variants in *TAOK3* encoding the serine/threonine-protein kinase	Correlated with increased acute postoperative pain and increased morphine requirements
Polymorphisms within a linkage disequilibrium block that spans 2q33.3-2q34	Strongly associated with the need for postoperative opioid analgesics, such as morphine and fentanyl, after painful surgery
Metabotropic glutamate receptors mGluR6 and mGluR8, nuclear receptor NR4A2, and cryptochrome 1	Evidence for involvement in heroin addiction
Calcium and potassium pathways genes	Multiple associations with opioid dependence

Data from Refs.[19–24]; and *From* Belfer I. Personalized pain medicine: pharmacogenetic testing for pain and opioid addiction. Pain Medicine News 2015. Available at: http://www.painmedicinenews.com/Review-Articles/Article/09-15/Personalized-Pain-Medicine-Pharmacogenetic-Testing-for-Pain-and-Opioid-Addiction/33480/ses=ogst. Accessed February 22, 2016; with permission.

Low Back Pain

Low back pain is highly prevalent and a leading cause of disability in the United States.[27] The causes are many, but degeneration of the spine and intervertebral discs is frequently blamed. Conventional scientific consensus says intervertebral disc degeneration and other spinal abnormalities are largely mechanical, but recent evidence has implicated genetic and biochemical mechanisms. In a study of 804 Chinese volunteers, aged 18 to 55, investigators found that a polymorphism—the Trp2 allele COL9A2 coding for α2 chain of collagen IX—is associated with a 4-fold increase in the risk of developing annular tears in people aged 30 to 39 years.[28] The molecule was associated with a 2.4-fold increase in the risk of developing degenerative disc disease and end-plate herniations in people aged 40 to 49 years. In addition, the presence of Trp2 predicted the severity of disc degeneration. The effect was more apparent in some age groups than in others. Boosting evidence that genetic risk factors vary among ethnicities, the Trp3 allele—shown to increase the risk of lumbar disc disease 3-fold in Finnish patients[29]—was absent in the Chinese population.

Finally, studies showed sex-specific genetic effects on pain when the same polymorphic allele predisposes one sex to more severe or more chronic pain and protects the other one. For example, female carriers of the minor allele of the A118G genotype in the *OPRM1* gene encoding the μ-opioid receptor (MOR) had 2.3 times as much sciatic pain as male carriers of this allele 12 months after lumbar disc herniation, demonstrating a slower recovery rate.[30]

Migraine

Migraine is more prevalent in women (17.1%) than in men (5.6%), and evidence points to an X-chromosome link, specifically at the locus of chromosome Xq24-28.[31,32] High anxiety and certain types of migraines have shown an association with the short (s) allele of the serotonin transporter gene 5HTTLPR polymorphism.[33] Several genome-wide association studies in migraine successfully identified at least 7 novel significantly contributing loci, located on chromosome 8q22.1, 2q37.1, 12q13.3, and 1p36.32.[34] Migraine with and without aura shares some genetic mechanisms but also may have separate genetic control.[35,36] Recent findings may further explain the observation that migraine with aura has female prevalence, whereas migraine without aura has male prevalence, reflecting sex-biased or even sex-antagonistic gene effects observed in general pain conditions.[37]

Fibromyalgia

FM is characterized by diffuse musculoskeletal pain and generalized tender points. It affects approximately 2% of the general population, and women are more susceptible than men.[38] Studies show FM to be more prevalent within families than in the general population[39,40]; however, the problem of isolating environmental and genetic factors continues. Some evidence exists that FM is an autosomal-dominant disorder.[41] An association of a gene for FM with human leukocyte antigen has been reported[42] and is further supported by research conducted in 40 multicase families with FM.[43] The T102C polymorphism of the *5-HT2A* serotonin receptor gene may contribute to nociception in FM, although a link has not been established in FM etiology. An investigation of the T102C allele found that FM patients exhibited a decrease in T/T and an increase in T/C and C/C genotypes when compared with healthy controls.[44] The pain scores for the T/T genotype were significantly higher than for T/C or C/C polymorphisms.

Several disorders associated with FM have similar symptoms and also appear to have a similar neuropathology. A large population-based study using the Swedish

Twin Registry determined that genetic factors contribute to the co-occurrence of FM with psychiatric disorders, including major depression, generalized anxiety disorder, and eating disorders.[45] Significant co-occurrences were found between FM and chronic fatigue, joint pain, depressive symptoms, and irritable bowel syndrome,[45] and yet another functional pain condition consists of temporomandibular joint disorders.[46] Several genes have been reported contributing to this family of painful diseases, including the serotonin transporter gene (SLC6A4),[47–49] interleukin-1 receptor antagonist (IL1RN) and melanocortin-1 receptor (MC1R) genes,[50] cytokine genes (IL6 and TNF-α),[51] and catechol-O-methyltransferase gene (COMT).[52–55] These complex medical conditions are often associated with a mosaic of motor, autonomic, neuroendocrine, and sleep abnormalities with research potential to understand the biological mechanisms that contribute to pain in these patients and may be affected by genetic polymorphism.[46]

Hereditary Pain Disorders

Interestingly, genes may contribute to both rare inherited and common pain disorders, reflecting their role in fundamental mechanisms of nociception and pain perception. For example, the SCN9A gene encoding for sodium channel Nav1.7 has loss-of-function rare mutations causing complete insensitivity to pain, gain-of-function rare mutations causing extreme pain phenotypes, and, finally, a common single-nucleotide polymorphism associated with 5 general pain conditions, including sciatica and low back pain.[12] A confirmation of the genetic association to perceived pain is found in 5 congenital disorders characterized by defects in normal sensation (**Box 1**).[56–60] Understanding genomic involvement with pain may lead to more precise pain therapies.

GENETICS OF ANALGESIA

Clinicians who treat pain have always known that the response to opioids varies widely among patients. Differences in bioavailability and pain stimuli explain some of this difference, but genetic makeup is likely a strong factor. Clinicians struggle with finding a consistent response to pain medications because of this tremendous interpatient response. There are several ways genetics influence drug response: through drug metabolism enzymes, drug transporters, opioid or other pain medication receptors, or structures involved in the perception and processing of pain.

Pharmacogenetics describes the effects of genetics on the pharmacokinetics (eg, drug absorption, distribution, metabolism, and excretion) and pharmacodynamics (through receptor activity, receptor binding affinity, and receptor density) of drugs.[61]

Box 1
Congenital disorders characterized by defects in normal pain processing

Congenital insensitivity to pain with anhidrosis

Familial dysautonomia (also called Riley-Day syndrome or hereditary sensory and autonomic neuropathy III)

Lesch-Nyhan syndrome

Tourette syndrome

De Lange syndrome

Data from Refs.[56–60]

What follows is a consideration of research involving certain genetic polymorphisms and their association with increased or reduced drug sensitivity.

Cytochrome P450 2D6 Gene

Among the most studied factors in drug metabolism is the CYP2D6, one of the cytochrome P450 (CYP) enzymes, which are a superfamily of drug-metabolizing enzymes that have shown variations in large populations.[62,63] Researchers have described more than 75 CYP2D6 alleles,[62] and further study has found that patients can be classified as poor metabolizers, intermediate metabolizers, extensive metabolizers, and ultrarapid metabolizers based on the number of CYP2D6 functional alleles.[64,65] Polymorphism of this gene helps explain tremendous individual differences in opioid requirements. Research has uncovered notable differences in the frequencies of alleles among different nations and ethnic groups.[64,66,67] Close to 29% of people in parts of East Africa may have multiple copies of CYP2D6, whereas the pattern is rare in Northern Europeans.[66] In fact, CYP2D6 gene duplication has been shown to occur in less than 2.6% of Caucasians.[67]

COMT

COMT metabolizes catecholamines and is important for dopaminergic and adrenergic/noradrenergic neurotransmission. A common polymorphism at amino acid position 158 (Val158Met) has been shown to impact human pain response.[68] Individuals with a homozygous methionine-158 genotype showed diminished regional μ-opioid system response to pain when compared with heterozygotes and also demonstrated higher sensory and affective ratings of pain. Patients with cancer with the Met/Met genotype also have shown a lower need for morphine compared with a Val/Val expression.[69]

OPRM1 118G

The MOR encoded by genetic locus OPRM1 is a prime site of action for endogenous opioid peptides and, thus, of interest to genetic investigators. Laboratory and clinical evidence has shown increased opioid requirements in patients with the OPRM1 118G polymorphism.[70–72] Of 120 patients who underwent total knee arthroplasty, patients who were 118G homozygotes consumed significantly more morphine than did patients who were 118A homozygotes or heterozygotes.[71] A further study found significantly greater opioid consumption to achieve pain control in 118G homozygotes compared with 118A homozygotes for hysterectomy patients during the first 24 hours postsurgery.[72] As previously mentioned, this common functional polymorphism has a sex-specific effect, with evidence that women carrying two 118G alleles experienced twice as much pain as male carriers.[30]

COMT/OPRM1 Interactions

Research also indicates that COMT and OPRM1 alleles synergistically interact, affecting analgesia; furthermore, combined COMT and MOR gene polymorphisms affect morphine postoperative analgesia and central side effects.[73] Heterozygous patients with opioid receptor A118G and the COMT G1947A mutation consumed significantly less morphine in the postanesthetic recovery room and 48 hours after surgery, compared with homozygous patients of the A118 variant.[73] Both genes have additional functional variants that may further shape analgesic effects. For example, a novel single-nucleotide polymorphism encoding for alternative MOR isoform contributes to individual differences in opiate response.[74] Furthermore, COMT haplotypes associated with great differences in enzymatic activity may predict analgesia with ββ-blockers in patients with chronic musculoskeletal pain.[75] Thus, common variants in these and other genes may influence analgesia independently or in combination with each other.

Melanocortin-1 Receptor Gene

The MC1R gene variants offer additional interesting evidence of the potential for highly targeted analgesia based on sex and other differences. There is evidence that women, more than men, respond to κ-induced analgesia,[76] which is mediated by the MC1R.[77] Women carrying 2 nonfunctional alleles displayed greater pentazocine (κ agonist) analgesic response than women with one or no such alleles, or men.[77] Furthermore, 75% of individuals with red hair and pale skin phenotypes carry 2 or more inactivating variants of the MC1R.[16]

JOINING THE GENETICS OF PAIN AND ANALGESIA FOR CLINICAL UTILITY

The variability in clinical effect among patients based on genotype emphasizes the need to perform pharmacogenetic assessments in patients, perhaps leading to the concept of "pharmacogenetic-based dose adaptation."[78]

The Spectrum of Medication Response

The opioid dose required for analgesia will be affected by genotype variants. One dose does not fit all. The categorization of opioid responders suggests a spectrum of possible responses after the same doses from analgesia to lack of efficacy to toxicity. For example, genotyping for CYP2D6 has resulted in work that suggests ultrarapid CYP2D6 metabolizers may possess enhanced endogenous pain-modulating mechanisms, lessening their requirements for postoperative morphine.[79] The ultrarapid phenotype also has been associated with faster analgesia but higher μ-opioid-related toxicity after tramadol[80] and oxycodone[81] administration. Conversely, poor metabolizers show reduced analgesia after codeine[82] and tramadol.[83]

Furthermore, poor metabolism of opioids could compromise the interpretations of urine drug testing administered to ensure compliance with opioid therapy. If genotyping were to reveal poor or ultrarapid opioid metabolizers, clinicians may find quantitative urine drug testing useful in assessing whether patients are consuming their prescriptions as directed.

Initiating Methadone: A Clinical Scenario

One clinical scenario that presents difficulty lies in initiating doses of methadone for pain. The Centers for Disease Control and Prevention reports that methadone is responsible for about one-third of opioid-related prescription drug deaths but represents only about 2% of all opioids prescribed.[84] The US Substance Abuse and Mental Health Services Administration cites as contributory the accumulation of methadone to a toxic level during initiation for pain therapy or addiction treatment because of an overestimation of tolerance and lack of consideration for methadone's long, variable half-life.[85] Because many deaths from methadone occur within the first few weeks of initiating therapy, poor methadone metabolism in a subset of patients may well be a factor.

The CYP enzyme system is a key player in methadone metabolism, and research is aimed at discovering which isoenzymes have the most influence. Although its metabolism is complex, methadone appears to be metabolized mainly by CYP2B6.[86,87] Testing for this isoenzyme may help identify who is at risk for slow metabolism and, therefore, toxicity from drug accumulation.

Adverse Drug Reactions

Genetic variations that impact a patient's drug sensitivity can lead to adverse reactions, toxicity, or therapeutic failure.[7] Of 27 drugs frequently cited in adverse drug reaction studies, 59% are metabolized by at least one enzyme with a variant allele known to cause poor metabolism.[88] That compares with 7% to 22% of randomly selected drugs. Tailoring therapy based on each individual's genotype should increase therapeutic effectiveness and minimize adverse effects.

SUMMARY

Each person carries his or her own genetic imprint for the risk of more severe or more chronic pain, pain perception, and response to analgesics. The environment may significantly influence how this genetic profile is expressed. Recent progress in genetic research indicates multiple gene-gene and gene × environment interactions that influence pain and analgesia as well common pathways among painful diseases. Studies of genetic polymorphisms linked to pain syndromes and medication metabolism herald a fresh therapeutic approach based on genotype with targeted analgesia and fewer side effects. However, genome-wide association studies are needed to complete a pain genome puzzle, identify full genetic signatures for pain and analgesia, and help genetic testing become a widespread part of clinical practice.

ACKNOWLEDGMENTS

Beth Dove of Dove Medical Communications, LLC, Salt Lake City, Utah, provided medical writing and manuscript review for this article.

REFERENCES

1. McClearn GE. Nature and nurture: interaction and coaction. Am J Med Genet B Neuropsychiatr Genet 2004;124B(1):124–30.
2. Young EE, Lariviere WR, Belfer I. Genetic basis of pain variability: recent advances. J Med Genet 2012;49(1):1–9.
3. Belfer I, Wu T, Kingman A, et al. Candidate gene studies of human pain mechanisms: methods for optimizing choice of polymorphisms and sample size. Anesthesiology 2004;100(6):1562–72.
4. Mogil JS, Wilson SG, Bon K, et al. Heritability of nociception I: responses of 11 inbred mouse strains on 12 measures of nociception. Pain 1999;80(1–2): 67–82.
5. Lariviere WR, Wilson SG, Laughlin TM, et al. Heritability of nociception. III. Genetic relationships among commonly used assays of nociception and hypersensitivity. Pain 2002;97(1–2):75–86.
6. Seltzer Z, Wu T, Max MB, et al. Mapping a gene for neuropathic pain-related behavior following peripheral neurectomy in the mouse. Pain 2001;93(2): 101–6.
7. Stamer UM, Stüber F. The pharmacogenetics of analgesia. Expert Opin Pharmacother 2007;8(14):2235–45.
8. Gilbert SC. Developmental biology. 6th edition. Sunderland (MA): Sinauer Associates; 2000. Available at: http://www.ncbi.nlm.nih.gov/books/NBK10023/. Accessed February 15, 2016.
9. Stranger BE, Stahl EA, Raj T. Progress and promise of genome-wide association studies for human complex trait genetics. Genetics 2011;187(2):367–83.

10. Belfer I. Personalized pain medicine: pharmacogenetic testing for pain and opioid addiction. Pain Medicine News 2015. Available at: http://www.painmedicinenews.com/Review-Articles/Article/09-15/Personalized-Pain-Medicine-Pharmacogenetic-Testing-for-Pain-and-Opioid-Addiction/33480/ses=ogst. Accessed February 22, 2016.

11. Fillingim RB, Kaplan L, Staud R, et al. The A118G single nucleotide polymorphism of the mu-opioid receptor gene (OPRM1) is associated with pressure pain sensitivity in humans. J Pain 2005;6(3):159–67.

12. Reimann F, Cox JJ, Belfer I, et al. Pain perception is altered by a nucleotide polymorphism in SCN9A. Proc Natl Acad Sci U S A 2010;107(11):5148–53.

13. Bortsov AV, Diatchenko L, McLean SA. Complex multilocus effects of catechol-O-methyltransferase haplotypes predict pain and pain interference 6 weeks after motor vehicle collision. Neuromolecular Med 2014;16(1):83–93.

14. Tegeder I, Costigan M, Griffin RS, et al. GTP cyclohydrolase and tetrahydrobiopterin regulate pain sensitivity and persistence. Nat Med 2006;12(11):1269–77.

15. Valdes AM, De Wilde G, Doherty SA, et al. The Ile585Val TRPV1 variant is involved in risk of painful knee osteoarthritis. Ann Rheum Dis 2011;70(9):1556–61.

16. Mogil JS, Ritchie J, Smith SB, et al. Melanocortin-1 receptor gene variants affect pain and mu-opioid analgesia in mice and humans. J Med Genet 2005;42(7):583–7.

17. Neely GG, Hess A, Costigan M, et al. A genome-wide Drosophila screen for heat nociception identifies α2δ3 as an evolutionarily conserved pain gene. Cell 2010;143(4):628–38.

18. Costigan M, Belfer I, Griffin RS, et al. Multiple chronic pain states are associated with a common amino acid-changing allele in KCNS1. Brain 2010;133(9):2519–27.

19. Peters MJ, Broer L, Willemen HL, et al. Genome-wide association study meta-analysis of chronic widespread pain: evidence for involvement of the 5p15.2 region. Ann Rheum Dis 2013;72(3):427–36.

20. Styrkarsdottir U, Thorleifsson G, Helgadottir HT, et al. Severe osteoarthritis of the hand associates with common variants within the ALDH1A2 gene and with rare variants at 1p31. Nat Genet 2014;46(5):498–502.

21. Cook-Sather SD, Li J, Goebel TK, et al. TAOK3, a novel genome-wide association study locus associated with morphine requirement and postoperative pain in a retrospective pediatric day surgery population. Pain 2014;155(9):1773–83.

22. Nishizawa D, Fukuda K, Kasai S, et al. Genome-wide association study identifies a potent locus associated with human opioid sensitivity. Mol Psychiatry 2014;19(1):55–62.

23. Nielsen DA, Ji F, Yuferov V, et al. Genotype patterns that contribute to increased risk for or protection from developing heroin addiction. Mol Psychiatry 2008;13(4):417–28.

24. Gelernter J, Kranzler HR, Sherva R, et al. Genome-wide association study of opioid dependence: multiple associations mapped to calcium and potassium pathways. Biol Psychiatry 2014;76(1):66–74.

25. MacGregor AJ, Andrew T, Sambrook PN, et al. Structural, psychological, and genetic influences on low back and neck pain: a study of adult female twins. Arthritis Rheum 2004;51(2):160–7.

26. Battié MC, Videman T, Levalahti E, et al. Heritability of low back pain and the role of disc degeneration. Pain 2007;131(3):272–80.

27. Institute of Medicine (US) Committee on Advancing Pain Research, Care, and Education. Relieving pain in America: a blueprint for transforming prevention,

care, education, and research. Washington (DC): National Academies Press (US); 2011. The National Academies Collection: Reports funded by National Institutes of Health.

28. Jim JJ, Noponen-Hietala N, Cheung KM, et al. The TRP2 allele of COL9A2 is an age-dependent risk factor for the development and severity of intervertebral disc degeneration. Spine (Phila Pa 1976) 2005;30(24):2735–42.

29. Paassilta P, Lohiniva J, Göring HH, et al. Identification of a novel common genetic risk factor for lumbar disk disease. JAMA 2001;285(14):1843–9.

30. Olsen MB, Jacobsen LM, Schistad EI, et al. Pain intensity the first year after lumbar disc herniation is associated with the A118G polymorphism in the opioid receptor mu 1 gene: evidence of a sex and genotype interaction. J Neurosci 2012; 32(29):9831–4.

31. Lipton RB, Bigal ME, Diamond M, et al. Migraine prevalence, disease burden, and the need for preventive therapy. Neurology 2007;68(5):343–9.

32. Nyholt DR, Curtain RP, Griffiths LR. Familial typical migraine: significant linkage and localization of a gene to Xq24-28. Hum Genet 2000;107(1):18–23.

33. Gonda X, Rihmer Z, Juhasz G, et al. High anxiety and migraine are associated with the s allele of the 5HTTLPR gene polymorphism. Psychiatry Res 2007; 149(1–3):261–6.

34. Tan MS, Jiang T, Tan L, et al. Genome-wide association studies in neurology. Ann Transl Med 2014;2(12):124.

35. Silberstein SD, Dodick DW. Migraine genetics–a review: part I. Headache 2013; 53(8):1207–17.

36. Silberstein SD, Dodick DW. Migraine genetics: part II. Headache 2013;53(8): 1218–29.

37. Belfer I, Segall SK, Lariviere WR, et al. Pain modality- and sex-specific effects of COMT genetic functional variants. Pain 2013;154(8):1368–76.

38. Chakrabarty S, Zoorob R. Fibromyalgia. Am Fam Physician 2007;76(2):247–54.

39. Arnold LM, Hudson JI, Hess EV, et al. Family study of fibromyalgia. Arthritis Rheum 2004;50(3):944–52.

40. Buskila D, Neumann L, Hazanov I, et al. Familial aggregation in the fibromyalgia syndrome. Semin Arthritis Rheum 1996;26(3):605–11.

41. Pellegrino MJ, Waylonis GW, Sommer A. Familial occurrence of primary fibromyalgia. Arch Phys Med Rehabil 1989;70(1):61–3.

42. Burda CD, Cox FR, Osborne P. Histocompatability antigens in the fibrositis (fibromyalgia) syndrome. Clin Exp Rheumatol 1986;4(4):355–8.

43. Yunus MB, Khan MA, Rawlings KK, et al. Genetic linkage analysis of multicase families with fibromyalgia syndrome. J Rheumatol 1999;26(2):408–12.

44. Bondy B, Spaeth M, Offenbaecher M, et al. The T102C polymorphism of the 5-HT2A-receptor gene in fibromyalgia. Neurobiol Dis 1999;6(5):433–9.

45. Kato K, Sullivan P, Evengård B, et al. Chronic widespread pain and its comorbidities: a population-based study. Arch Intern Med 2006;166(15):1649–54.

46. Diatchenko L, Fillingim RB, Smith SB, et al. The phenotypic and genetic signatures of common musculoskeletal pain conditions. Nat Rev Rheumatol 2013; 9(6):340–50.

47. Ablin JN, Cohen H, Buskila D. Mechanisms of disease: genetics of fibromyalgia. Nat Clin Pract Rheumatol 2006;2(12):671–8.

48. Narita M, Nishigami N, Narita N, et al. Association between serotonin transporter gene polymorphism and chronic fatigue syndrome. Biochem Biophys Res Commun 2003;311(2):264–6.

49. Herken H, Erdal E, Mutlu N, et al. Possible association of temporomandibular joint pain and dysfunction with a polymorphism in the serotonin transporter gene. Am J Orthod Dentofacial Orthop 2001;120(3):308–13.

50. Foster DC, Sazenski TM, Stodgell CJ. Impact of genetic variation in interleukin-1 receptor antagonist and melanocortin-1 receptor genes on vulvar vestibulitis syndrome. J Reprod Med 2004;49(7):503–9.

51. Barkhordari E, Rezaei N, Ansaripour B, et al. Proinflammatory cytokine gene polymorphisms in irritable bowel syndrome. J Clin Immunol 2010;30(1):74–9.

52. Cohen H, Neumann L, Glazer Y, et al. The relationship between a common catechol-O-methyltransferase (COMT) polymorphism val(158) met and fibromyalgia. Clin Exp Rheumatol 2009;27(5 Suppl 56):S51–6.

53. Barbosa FR, Matsuda JB, Mazucato M, et al. Influence of catechol-O-methyltransferase (COMT) gene polymorphisms in pain sensibility of Brazilian fibromialgia patients. Rheumatol Int 2012;32(2):427–30.

54. Diatchenko L, Slade GD, Nackley AG, et al. Genetic basis for individual variations in pain perception and the development of a chronic pain condition. Hum Mol Genet 2005;14(1):135–43.

55. Karling P, Danielsson Å, Wikgren M, et al. The relationship between the val158met catechol-O-methyltransferase (COMT) polymorphism and irritable bowel syndrome. PLoS One 2011;6(3):e18035.

56. Berkovitch M, Copeliovitch L, Tauber T, et al. Hereditary insensitivity to pain with anhidrosis. Pediatr Neurol 1998;19(3):227–9.

57. Blumenfeld A, Slaugenhaupt SA, Axelrod FB, et al. Localization of the gene for familial dysautonomia on chromosome 9 and definition of DNA markers for genetic diagnosis. Nat Genet 1993;4(2):160–4.

58. Shapira J, Zilberman Y, Becker A. Lesch-Nyhan syndrome: a nonextracting approach to prevent mutilation. Spec Care Dentist 1985;5(5):210–2.

59. Lowe O. Tourette's syndrome: management of oral complications. ASDC J Dent Child 1986;53(6):456–60.

60. Shear CS, Nyhan WL, Kirman BH, et al. Self-mutilative behavior as a feature of the de Lange syndrome. J Pediatr 1971;78(3):506–9.

61. Somogyi AA, Barratt DT, Coller JK. Pharmacogenetics of opioids. Clin Pharmacol Ther 2007;81(3):429–44.

62. Weinshilboum R. Inheritance and drug response. N Engl J Med 2003;348(6): 529–37.

63. Nelson DR. The cytochrome p450 homepage. Hum Genomics 2009;4(1):59–65.

64. McGraw J, Waller D. Cytochrome P450 variations in different ethnic populations. Expert Opin Drug Metab Toxicol 2012;8(3):371–82.

65. Johansson I, Lundqvist E, Bertilsson L, et al. Inherited amplification of an active gene in the cytochrome P450 CYP2D locus as a cause of ultrarapid metabolism of debrisoquine. Proc Natl Acad Sci U S A 1993;90:11825–9.

66. Aklillu E, Persson I, Bertilsson L, et al. Frequent distribution of ultrarapid metabolizers of debrisoquine in an Ethiopian population carrying duplicated and multi-duplicated functional CYP2D6 alleles. J Pharmacol Exp Ther 1996;278:441–6.

67. Sachse C, Brockmöller J, Bauer S, et al. Cytochrome P450 2D6 variants in a Caucasian population: allele frequencies and phenotypic consequences. Am J Hum Genet 1997;60(2):284–95.

68. Zubieta JK, Heitzeg MM, Smith YR, et al. COMT val158met genotype affects mu-opioid neurotransmitter responses to a pain stressor. Science 2003;299(5610): 1240–3.

69. Rakvåg TT, Klepstad P, Baar C, et al. The Val158Met polymorphism of the human catechol-O-methyltransferase (COMT) gene may influence morphine requirements in cancer pain patients. Pain 2005;116(1–2):73–8.

70. Klepstad P, Rakvåg TT, Kaasa S, et al. The 118 A > G polymorphism in the human mu-opioid receptor gene may increase morphine requirements in patients with pain caused by malignant disease. Acta Anaesthesiol Scand 2004;48(10): 1232–9.

71. Chou WY, Yang LC, Lu HF, et al. Association of mu-opioid receptor gene polymorphism (A118G) with variations in morphine consumption for analgesia after total knee arthroplasty. Acta Anaesthesiol Scand 2006;50(7):787–92.

72. Chou WY, Wang CH, Liu PH, et al. Human opioid receptor A118G polymorphism affects intravenous patient-controlled analgesia morphine consumption after total abdominal hysterectomy. Anesthesiology 2006;105(2):334–7.

73. Kolesnikov Y, Gabovits B, Levin A, et al. Combined catechol-O-methyltransferase and mu-opioid receptor gene polymorphisms affect morphine postoperative analgesia and central side effects. Anesth Analg 2011;112(2):448–53.

74. Shabalina SA, Zaykin DV, Gris P, et al. Expansion of the human mu-opioid receptor gene architecture: novel functional variants. Hum Mol Genet 2009;18(6): 1037–51.

75. Tchivileva IE, Lim PF, Smith SB, et al. Effect of catechol-O-methyltransferase polymorphism on response to propranolol therapy in chronic musculoskeletal pain: a randomized, double-blind, placebo-controlled, crossover pilot study. Pharmacogenet Genomics 2010;20(4):239–48.

76. Gear RW, Miaskowski C, Gordon NC, et al. Kappa-opioids produce significantly greater analgesia in women than in men. Nat Med 1996;2(11):1248–50.

77. Mogil JS, Wilson SG, Chesler EJ, et al. The melanocortin-1 receptor gene mediates female-specific mechanisms of analgesia in mice and humans. Proc Natl Acad Sci U S A 2003;100(8):4867–72.

78. Lötsch J, Geisslinger G. Current evidence for a genetic modulation of the response to analgesics. Pain 2006;121(1–2):1–5.

79. Candiotti KA, Yang Z, Rodriguez Y, et al. The impact of CYP2D6 genetic polymorphisms on postoperative morphine consumption. Pain Med 2009;10(5):799–805.

80. Kirchheiner J, Keulen JT, Bauer S, et al. Effects of the CYP2D6 gene duplication on the pharmacokinetics and pharmacodynamics of tramadol. J Clin Psychopharmacol 2008;28(1):78–83.

81. de Leon J, Dinsmore L, Wedlund P. Adverse drug reactions to oxycodone and hydrocodone in CYP2D6 ultrarapid metabolizers. J Clin Psychopharmacol 2003;23(4):420–1.

82. Brousseau DC, McCarver DG, Drendel AL, et al. The effect of CYP2D6 polymorphisms on the response to pain treatment for pediatric sickle cell pain crisis. J Pediatr 2007;150(6):623–6.

83. Stamer UM, Lehnen K, Höthker F, et al. Impact of CYP2D6 genotype on postoperative tramadol analgesia. Pain 2003;105(1–2):231–8.

84. Centers for Disease Control and Prevention (CDC). Vital signs: Prescription painkiller overdoses: use and abuse of methadone as a painkiller. 2012. Available at: http://www.cdc.gov/vitalsigns/MethadoneOverdoses. Accessed February 12, 2016.

85. Center for Substance Abuse Treatment. Methadone-associated mortality: report of a national assessment. Rockville (MD): Center for Substance Abuse Treatment, Substance Abuse and Mental Health Services Administration; 2004. CSAT Publication No. 28-03.

86. Kharasch ED, Regina KJ, Blood J, et al. Methadone pharmacogenetics: CYP2B6 polymorphisms determine plasma concentrations, clearance, and metabolism. Anesthesiology 2015;123(5):1142–53.
87. Dobrinas M, Crettol S, Oneda B, et al. Contribution of CYP2B6 alleles in explaining extreme (S)-methadone plasma levels: a CYP2B6 gene resequencing study. Pharmacogenet Genomics 2013;23(2):84–93.
88. Phillips KA, Veenstra DL, Oren E, et al. Potential role of pharmacogenomics in reducing adverse drug reactions: a systematic review. JAMA 2001;286(18): 2270–9.

Pharmacogenomics in Psychiatric Practice

Rif S. El-Mallakh, MD[a],*, R. Jeannie Roberts, MD[b], Peggy L. El-Mallakh, PhD[c], Lillian Jan Findlay, PhD[c], Kristen K. Reynolds, PhD[d]

KEYWORDS

- Psychiatric pharmacogenomics • Pharmacogenomic testing • Antidepressants
- Antipsychotics • 2D6 • *CYP2D6* • *SLC6A4* • *OPRM1*

KEY POINTS

- Growth in psychopharmacogenomics is occurring in specific gene variants that predict specific response/nonresponse to specific agents.
- Some of the important genes include *CYP2D6, SLC6A4, HTR1A, HTR1A, COMT, MTHFR, OPRM1,* and *OPRD1.*
- Psychiatric pharmacogenomics is becoming an established clinical procedure.

Pharmacogenomics in psychiatry is in early phase of clinical application and acceptance. There are now data available that demonstrate that pharmacogenomic testing is associated with better outcomes and reduced complications in depressed patients.[1,2] Evidence continues to accumulate for additional genetic variants and improved clinical and economic outcomes. This article reviews the current state-of-the-art application of psychiatric pharmacogenomics.

Disclosure Statement: Dr R.S. El-Mallakh receives research funding from the National Institute of Mental Health (NIMH-R42 MH091997), the State of Kentucky, Teva, PsychNostics, and Merck. He is a speaker for Lundbeck, Merck, Otsuka, Sunovion, and Takeda. Dr K.K. Reynolds is an employee of PGXL, a company that performs pharmacogenomic testing. Drs L.J. Findlay, R.J. Roberts, and P.L. El-Mallakh do not have conflicts of interest to report.
 ^a Mood Disorders Research Program, Department of Psychiatry and Behavioral Sciences, University of Louisville HealthCare OutPatient Center, University of Louisville School of Medicine, 401 East Chestnut Street, Suite 610, Louisville, KY 40202, USA; ^b Department of Psychiatry and Behavioral Sciences, University of Louisville HealthCare OutPatient Center, University of Louisville Hospital, University of Louisville School of Medicine, 401 East Chestnut Street, Suite 610, Louisville, KY 40202, USA; ^c Graduate Psychiatric-Mental Health Nursing Program, University of Kentucky College of Nursing, University of Kentucky, 547 College of Nursing Building, Lexington, KY 40536-0232, USA; ^d PGXL Laboratories, Department of Pathology, University of Louisville School of Medicine, University of Louisville, 201 East Jefferson Street, Suite 309, Louisville, KY 40202, USA
* Corresponding author.
E-mail address: rselma01@louisville.edu

Clin Lab Med 36 (2016) 507–523
http://dx.doi.org/10.1016/j.cll.2016.05.001
0272-2712/16/$ – see front matter © 2016 Elsevier Inc. All rights reserved.

Psychiatric pharmacogenomics had its genesis in the understanding of avoidance of toxicity with the older tricyclic antidepressants.[3] These early antidepressant agents were clearly effective, for example,[4] but carried the liability of problematic or intolerable adverse effects (AEs) and potentially fatal cardiotoxicity.[5–7] Despite documentation of genetic variants that alter tricyclic metabolism and identify at risk patients,[8] the predominate approach was to use therapeutic drug level monitoring.[9] With the introduction of the safer serotonin-reuptake inhibiting antidepressants, the focus has shifted to predicting efficacy, particularly in treatment-resistant patients.[10]

Nonetheless, work in understanding the genetic basis of drug response and experience of AEs has continued. In other fields of medicine, personalized medicine has clearly altered the outcome of treatment,[11,12] but in psychiatry, the field is still in its infancy. Development of pharmacogenomic targets has been delayed due to relatively small effect sizes that may not be evident in large screening studies.[13] One of the limitations to greater application of genomic testing in psychiatric patients is concern regarding the cost-effectiveness of the testing. It seems clear that subjects with P450 or other predisposing gene variants are less likely to achieve remission and more likely to be responsible for high resource utilization,[14] and that knowledge of pharmacogenomic profile improves treatment outcome.[15] Most available antidepressant agents work by modulating activity of the biogenic amines: serotonin, dopamine, norepinephrine, melatonin, and histamine. Universally, they share similar rates of efficacy in that approximately a third respond to placebo, a third respond to the medication, and a third do not respond. The high rate of nonresponse creates a situation in which many patients are given a serial train of antidepressant agents over time.[16,17] In addition to the suffering experienced by many of these individuals, this process of multiple switches increases the cost[18] and reduces patient confidence and increases likelihood of patient dropout from treatment.[19,20] These issues can be addressed, in part, by attempts to personalize treatments to improve outcomes.[21,22] Individual studies, meta-analyses,[23] and pharmacoeconomic modeling,[22] all suggest that use of pharmacogenomic testing in treatment-resistant major depressive disorder is cost-effective. Furthermore, pharmacogenomic testing is positively perceived by young clinicians and scientists.[24]

Pharmacogenomics in psychiatry can be divided into genetic markers that predict AEs (mainly P450 genetic variants) and genetic markers that predict positive response to a particular medication (specific markers).

METHODS

Searches were performed with PubMed and Google Scholar by using searches combining "pharmacogenomics" with "schizophrenia," "psychosis," "major depression," "bipolar," "alcohol abuse," "opioid abuse," "cocaine abuse," "methamphetamine abuse," and "cannabis abuse." Only replicated studies were incorporated into this review. Many more potential markers have been reported in the literature, so limiting the review to replicated markers was necessary. Thus, this is not a comprehensive review, but a much more targeted review compilation of the literature.

P450 MARKERS

There are approximately 60 P450 genes that code for proteins that are involved in either detoxification of exogenous compounds or physiologic metabolism of endogenous compounds. P450 proteins that are aimed at endogenous compounds generally are involved in the biosynthesis or catabolism of retinoids, or fatty compounds, such as steroids, prostaglandins, and fatty acids.[25] Because they are needed for normal physiologic activity, they are generally conserved and distributed in multiple tissues. One such example is P450 3A4, which due to its reduced variability has fewer clinically relevant variants (**Table 1**).[26] P450 proteins that are intended to detoxify xenobiotic compounds are distributed in the liver and epithelial tissues and tend to be more variable.[25] These enzymes have broad substrate specificity and will oxidize, reduce, or hydrolyze potentially toxic xenobiotic compounds to make them water-soluble so the kidney can eliminate them.[27] Collectively, all the P450 enzymes are responsible for metabolizing more than 90% of pharmaceuticals.[28] A large number of clinically significant variants have been identified (see **Table 1**).

In general, clinical phenotypes associated with P450 variants are divided into poor metabolizers, intermediate metabolizers, extensive metabolizers, and ultrarapid metabolizers. The extensive metabolizer designation generally refers to the wild-type or most common functional version of the gene. Patients classified as poor metabolizers generally have 2 copies of essentially nonfunctional alleles. Intermediate metabolizing patients have 1 good copy and 1 nonfunctional copy. Those designated as ultrarapid metabolizers generally have multiple copies of a functioning allele. Generally, patients who are poor or intermediate metabolizers will experience more

Table 1
Frequently tested genes, their function, and potentially problematic variants

Protein	Variants	Consequences
CYP2D6	*9, *10, *17, *29, *41 (or heterozygous with inactive variants below)	Intermediate metabolizers.
CYP2D6	*3, *4, *5 (deletion), *6, *7, *8, *11, *12, *14, *15	Poor metabolizers.
CYP2D6	Gene duplication *1, *2, *4, *6, *9, *10, *17, *29, *41	Ultrarapid metabolizers.
CYP2C19	*2, *3, *4, *5, *6, *7, *8, *9, *10	Poor metabolizers or intermediate metabolizers when heterozygous with *1.
CYP2C19	*17	Ultrarapid metabolizers.
CYP2C9	*2, *3, *4, *5, *6, *8, *11, *12	Poor metabolizers or Intermediate metabolizers when heterozygous with *1.
CYP3A4	*3, *17, *22	Poor metabolizers or intermediate metabolizers when heterozygous with *1.
SLC6A4 (serotonin transporter)	Short form or A > G polymorphism	Reduced response or increased side effects with serotoninergic antidepressants.
OPRM1 (mu-1 opioid receptor)	118A > G	GG (homozygous variant) genotype requires much higher opioid doses to achieve pain relief, and lower relapse rates into alcohol dependence with naltrexone treatment. AA genotype displays higher relapse rates with naltrexone treatment for alcohol dependence.

AEs with the pharmaceutical substrate, whereas ultrarapid metabolizers generally will not respond. Patients who are extensive metabolizers will generally have few AEs and will have an "average" response. Common substrates of P450 enzymes are shown in **Table 2.**

In addition to the basal rate of P450 enzyme activity, different enzymes can be induced or inhibited differently, based on their sequence. The most important of these is the CYP1A2*1F variant, which confers great inducibility of the 1A2 gene in the presence of cigarette smoke, greater than the level induced in subjects without this single nucleotide polymorphism (SNP).[29,30] This is an example of the potential complexity of such CYP450 variants.

Although there is ample evidence that P450 genotypes may partially predict medication response,[31] there are published reports that suggest the P450 genotypes may not be as predictive as believed.[32] However, these negative studies are designed for convenience and not to answer the specific research question addressed. A bigger issue is that variants related to disease susceptibility are much more powerful predictors of response and lack of AEs, and that is the current direction of research.[33]

MOOD DISORDERS
Treatment Outcome

SLC6A4
The serotonin transporter gene has garnered a fair amount of attention. It codes for the serotonin-reuptake pump: the same protein that must be inhibited by nearly all antidepressants. Initial studies revealed that individuals who have the "short form" (homozygous or heterozygous) of the serotonin transporter are more likely to become depressed in the setting of adversity.[34] Subsequent studies confirmed this relationship for Africans and Caucasians but not Asians.[35,36] "Short" refers to a 44 base-pair deletion in the promoter region of the gene.[37] Individuals with this deletion express fewer,[38] but functionally intact[39] serotonin-reuptake pumps in the synapse. In addition to increased likelihood for depression, individuals with the short form are less likely to respond, or have a delayed response, to antidepressants.[35,40] Additionally, these individuals were more likely to experience AEs when given an antidepressant.[41] People with bipolar illness and the short form, are more likely to experience rapid cycling when exposed to an antidepressant.[35] It has been suggested that the short form may also be responsible for the troubling phenomenon of tachyphylaxis: loss of efficacy of antidepressants with time.[35,42] A very different SNP in which an adenine is replaced with a guanine (usually designated L_G) has the same phenotype as the "short form."[43] When clinical laboratories test for the short form, they usually test for the L_G allele as well. The clinical implications of the short form are not clear due to ethnic variation. Among Caucasians, the short form/L_G predicts poorer antidepressant response and greater cost of care of treating major depression without gene testing.[36]

Catechol-O-methyltransferase
The catechol-O-methyltransferase (COMT) gene catalyzes the transfer of a methyl group from S-adenosylmethionine to the neurotransmitter catecholamines, dopamine, epinephrine, and norepinephrine. A polymorphism in which methionine, the 158th amino acid, is replaced with valine (Val/Val, rs4680) predicts poor response to all antidepressants, but particularly serotonin/norepinephrine reuptake inhibitors.[44–46]

Serotonin receptors, HTR2A, HTR1A, and HTR1B
HTR2A codes for the serotonin 2A postsynaptic receptor. In several large studies, the TT allele of the rs6313 SNP was associated with improvement to antidepressant

Table 2
The primary CYP metabolic pathway for common psychotropics

Agent	2D6	3A4	1A2	2C19	2C9	Non-P450 Enzyme
Antidepressants						
Amitriptyline (Elavil, Levate)	✔			✔		
Clomipramine (Anafranil)	✔			✔		
Citalopram/Escitalopram (Celexa/Lexapro)				✔		
Desipramine (Norpramin)	✔					
Desvenlafaxine (Pristiq)						✔
Doxepin (Sinequan)	✔			✔		
Duloxetine (Cymbalta)	✔		✔			
Fluoxetine (Prozac)	✔					
Fluvoxamine (Luvox)	✔					
Imipramine (Tofranil)	✔			✔		
Levomilnacipran (Fetzima, Dalcipran, Ixel, Toledomin)		✔				
Maprotiline (Ludiomil)	✔					
Mirtazapine (Remeron)	✔					
Nefazodone (Serzone)		✔				
Nortriptyline (Pamelor, Aventyl)	✔					
Paroxetine (Paxil)	✔					
Sertraline (Zoloft)				✔		
Trazadone (Desyrel)		✔				
Trimipramine (Surmontil)	✔			✔		
Venlafaxine (Effexor)	✔					
Vilazodone (Viibryd)		✔				
Vortioxetine (Brintellix)	✔					
Antipsychotics						
Aripiprazole (Abilify)	✔	✔				
Asenapine (Saphris)			✔			
Brexpiprazole (Rexulti)	✔	✔				
Chlorpromazine (Thorazine)	✔					
Clozapine (Clozaril, Fazaclo)			✔			
Haloperidol (Haldol)	✔					
Iloperidone (Fanapt)	✔					
Loxapine (Loxitane, Loxapac, Adasuve)	✔	✔	✔			
Lurasidone (Latuda)		✔				
Olanzapine (Zyprexa)			✔			
Quetiapine (Seroquel)		✔				
Paliperidone (Invega, Sustenna, Trinza)						✔
Perphenazine (Trilafon)	✔					
Risperidone (Risperdal, Consta)	✔					

(continued on next page)

Table 2
(continued)

Agent	2D6	3A4	1A2	2C19	2C9	Non-P450 Enzyme
Thioridazine (Mellaril)	✔					
Thiothixene (Navane)			✔			
Ziprasidone (Geodon)		✔				✔
Mood stabilizers						
Carbamazepine (Tegretol, Carbatrol, Equetro)		✔				
Diltiazem (Cardizem)		✔				
Lamotrigine (Lamictal)						✔
Nifedipine (Adalat)		✔				
Phenytoin (Dilantin)					✔	
Valproic acid (Depakote, Depakene)				✔		
Verapamil (Calan, Isoptin, Verelan)		✔				
Pain management						
Buprenorphine (Subutex, Suboxone)		✔				
Codeine	✔					
Hydrocodone	✔					
Methadone (the active R enantiomer)				✔		
Oxycodone	✔					
Tramadol	✔					
Other psychotropics						
Alprazolam (Xanax)		✔				
Amphetamine/dextroamphetamine (Adderall, Dexedrine) Lisdexamfetamine (Vyvanse)	✔					
Atomoxetine (Strattera)	✔					
Buspirone (Buspar)		✔				
Caffeine			✔			
Diazepam (Valium)				✔		
Gabapentin (Neurontin)						✔
Ketamine/Esketamine (Ketalar)		✔				
Ramelteon (Rozerem)			✔			
Suvorexant (Belsomra)		✔				
Zolpidem (Ambien)		✔				

Note: Agents not metabolized by P450 enzymes have least likelihood of having interindividual variation.

treatment.[47,48] *HTR1A* and *HTR1B* code for the serotonin receptors 5HT$_{1A}$ and 5HT$_{1B}$, respectively. Both are believed to act as presynaptic autoreceptors, and their down-regulation is believed to be important for serotonin-reuptake inhibiting antidepressants.[49] In 153 patients receiving citalopram in the Sequenced Treatment Alternatives to Relieve Depression (STAR*D) study, SNPs associated with overexpression of $5HT_{1A}$ and $5HT_{1B}$ predicted nonresponse or a delayed response to citalopram.[49]

Brain-derived neurotrophic factor

Brain-derived neurotrophic factor (BDNF) codes for a protein that promotes neuronal survival, and has been associated with treatment response in depression.[50] A polymorphism, rs6265 or Val66Met, has been associated with more severe depressive illness.[51] However, the findings that these same patients do less well with antidepressants has not be readily replicated.[52,53]

Potassium channel

Potassium channel, KCNK2, codes for a potassium channel that leaks potassium out of the cell to control resting membrane potential (http://www.ncbi.nlm.nih.gov/gene/3776). The channel can be controlled by multiple neurotransmitter signals (eg, serotonin and glutamate[54]) and will allow more potassium to leak out when the membrane is stretched, heated, or when the cytosol becomes more acidic (http://www.ncbi.nlm.nih.gov/gene/3776). Absence of the gene in animals results in resistance to developing depression in the setting of stress.[55] In a study of 1554 patients in the STAR*D study, SNP variants of KCNK2 were associated with treatment resistance to both citalopram and subsequent treatment steps (bupropion, or other serotoninergic antidepressants).[54]

ATP binding cassette subfamily B member 1 protein

The ATP binding cassette subfamily B member 1 protein (ABCB1) appears to play a role in the transport of antidepressants across membranes. Several SNPs have been associated with a better antidepressant response and increased side effects.[56–60] Because of its role in antidepressant transport, there is an interplay between plasma antidepressant levels and drug response, with optimal response when levels are maintained in the accepted therapeutic range.[58] Conversely, when patient gene testing results were incorporated into decision making, hospitalized depressed patients were discharged earlier if gene testing was performed and dose increased as a consequence of test results.[61]

FK506 binding protein 5

The FK506 binding protein 5 is coded for by FKBP5. It is involved in immunoregulation and basic cellular processes involving protein folding and trafficking, and it binds to the immunosuppressant FK506, hence the name. Individuals with depression and with the C-allele of the rs1360780 polymorphism generally responded better to antidepressants in structured settings with a small effect size.[62,63]

GNB3

GNB3 is a gene that codes for a beta subunit of signal transducing G protein. The rs5443 polymorphism (C825T) has been associated with increased likelihood of response and remission with serotonin-reuptake inhibiting antidepressants.[64]

PPP3CC

PPP3CC is the gamma isozyme of protein phosphatase 3, which is the catalytic subunit of calcineurin, a calcium-dependent, calmodulin-stimulated protein phosphatase involved in the downstream regulation of dopaminergic signal transduction. SNPs of this gene have been associated with antidepressant outcome in multiple studies.[48,65]

Methylenetetrahydrofolate reductase

Methylenetetrahydrofolate reductase (MTHFR) is required for the conversion of 5,10-methylenetetrahydrofolate to 5-methyltetrahydrofolate, which is a cosubstrate for homocysteine remethylation to methionine. The T variant of the C677T SNP (rs1801133) has been associated with an increased risk for depression.[66] Use of L-methylfolate supplementation (usually 15 mg per day), has been shown to augment the antidepressant response in poorly responsive patients, and the MTHFR C677T SNP has been believed to be important in this response[67,68] although direct evidence is suboptimal.[69]

PSYCHOSIS
Treatment Response

The dopamine D2 receptor (DRD2) is highly associated with antipsychotic response in patients with psychosis. It has also been associated with schizophrenia in genome-wide association studies.[70] The SNP most closely associated with the predisposition to schizophrenia is rs2514218, where a C has replaced a T, approximately 47 kb upstream from DRD2. This same SNP also appears to predict antipsychotic response across multiple different agents.[71–73] Another polymorphism of the DRD2 (rs1079597), was associated with improvement in negative symptoms in 125 patients with schizophrenia receiving the antipsychotic amisulpride for 12 weeks.[74]

The SULT4A1 is a highly conserved gene that codes for a brain-specific sulfotransferase that is believed to be involved in the metabolism of neurotransmitters.[75] Two SNPs, rs138060 and rs138097, were significantly associated with greater symptom burden and reduced cognition, respectively.[76] In the Clinical Antipsychotic Trials of Intervention Effectiveness (CATIE) trial, patients with schizophrenia carrying a specific haplotype, designated SULT4A1-1, were more symptomatic and had greater improvement with reduced risk for hospitalization than patients lacking the haplotype when treated with olanzapine.[77,78] However, across several other trials, this finding could not be reproduced.[79]

The dopamine D1 receptor (DRD1) has been investigated, but after initial suggestive evidence that a particular polymorphism may be associated with treatment outcome (s4532),[80] accumulated data suggested no association.[81]

Similar contradictory data were described for SNPs within the neuronal adhesion molecule coded for by neurexin 1 (NRXN1). In a small placebo-controlled study, rs12467557 and rs10490162[82] were associated with greater response to antipsychotics, but this could not be replicated with the CATIE trial sample.[83]

Polymorphisms and Neurocognition

A growing body of research suggests that pharmacogenomics can guide the clinical decision making related to clinical issues that have historically plagued clinicians who prescribe antipsychotics in the treatment of schizophrenia. Recent research suggests that genetic polymorphisms are linked to treatment refractoriness,[32,84] and antipsychotic weight gain.[85]

There is some evidence that polymorphisms in COMT (the Met/Met genotype rs4680 [Val158Met]) and MTHFR (the CC genotype) may be associated with cognitive deficits in patients with psychosis.[86,87] There is also evidence that the rs6295 polymorphism (G/G subjects) of the serotonin 1A receptor (HTR1A) is associated with improvement in cognition with treatment with clozapine.[86]

Metabolic Disturbances

Research indicates that polymorphisms of several genes are linked to antipsychotic weight gain, including orexin,[88] protein kinase C-amp-dependent regulatory type II beta (PRKAR2B),[89] and *MTHFR*.[90] An SNP of *MTHFR* (rs1801131, AC or CC, not AA) may predict which patients who have gained weight might lose it when switched to aripiprazole or ziprasidone.[91]

Fonseka and colleagues[85] suggest that genetic variations in interleukin (IL)-1beta, IL-2, IL-6, and BDNF play a role in antipsychotic weight gain. Similarly, Roffeei and colleagues[92] reported that among patients with schizophrenia receiving antipsychotic treatment in Malaysia, polymorphisms of rs9939609 of the *FTO* gene significantly increased risk for metabolic syndrome (odds ratio [OR] 1.73, 95% confidence interval [CI] 1.07–2.78, P = .026). However, they found that 2 polymorphisms were protective against metabolic syndrome, including rs1137101 of the *LEPR* gene (OR 0.47, 95% CI 0.28–0.80, P = .005), and the re1801133 of the *MTHFR* gene (OR 0.59, 95% CI 0.35–0.99, P = .049).[92] Among Han Chinese, several SNPs of the serotonin-reuptake pump (*SLC6A4*) have been identified as predisposing patients to weight gain with risperidone.[93] However, the effect of one SNP (rs3813034) was greater than all the others.[93]

SUBSTANCE USE DISORDERS

There is a continuing search for genetic markers with variants that are related to different substance use disorders that may point the way to medications that would target the markers in a way to nullify the effects or reduce the use of the specific abused drug while reducing the toxicity and adverse reactions of the medications. Although many genetic markers associated with different disorders have been postulated and are currently being studied, there are few medication treatments that target these genes at this time.

Alcohol Use Disorders

Naltrexone
Genes associated with naltrexone treatment for ethanol dependence are *OPRM1*, *OPRD1*, and *OPRK1*. The most common studied gene believed affected by naltrexone is *OPRM1* with an allele variant change from asparagine (Asn) to aspartate (Asp) (amino acid substitution, Asp40Asn, or 118A > G). Individuals with this SNP have symptoms of altered alcohol subjective effects, and treatment with naltrexone alters the response to cortisol by increasing that response.[94] The frequency of this gene in the overall population is low: Caucasian individuals have approximately 20% ASP40, African American individuals with 5%, and Asian individuals as high as 50%. Consequently, population-wide studies that do not genotype participants show no differences between naltrexone and placebo.[95,96] Studies that specifically investigate the effect of Asn40Asp find increased rates of response to naltrexone.[97–99]

Acamprosate
The *GRIN2B* gene product is believed to be the target of acamprosate. Subjects with a minor A variant had slightly more significant time to relapse than their peers.[100]

Stimulant (Cocaine, Methamphetamine) Use Disorders

Disulfiram
Subjects with the Ala222Val SNP (CT or TT) of the *MTHFR* gene appeared to be less likely to relapse into cocaine use when treated with disulfiram compared with subjects with the CC genotype.[101] The Ala222Val variant is most common in people with an African heritage (78%), and less common in Caucasian (46%) and Hispanic (31%) individuals.[102]

Opioid Use Disorders

Naltrexone

Naltrexone is an opioid antagonist. It prevents opioids from activating the mu-opioid receptors. It binds more tightly than heroin, morphine, or methadone.[103] Persons with 1 or 2 variant alleles (C17T and A118G) of the mu-opioid receptor (*OPRM1*) have been shown to have higher basal levels of the stress hormone, cortisol.[104] Stress hormones have been related to measures of recovery from addiction, including time to relapse. Persons with these variants may respond better to naltrexone.[105]

Buprenorphine

This drug is a partial agonist at the mu-opioid receptor site and an antagonist at the kappa-opioid receptor site. As with methadone, it has high affinity for the receptor and a slow dissociation that makes it effective for treatment of opioid dependence. Response to this medication has been associated with the delta-opioid receptor gene, *OPRD1*. African American men treated with buprenorphine were more likely to have positive urine tests; that is, less likely to benefit, if they had the CC variant of the SNP rs678849.[106] This was not true for European Americans, nor for either sample in the methadone group.[106] A similar study found that women with the AA or AG genotype at rs581111 or rs529520, of *OPRD1,* had significantly worse outcome than those with CC.[107] Men were not significantly different in any comparison.[107]

THE FUTURE OF PHARMACOGENOMICS IN PSYCHIATRY

Promising approaches toward potential opportunities for genetic testing have been proposed in the literature. For example, Verbelen and Lewis[108] suggested that pharmacogenomic testing can be developed to identify risk for clozapine-induced agranulocytosis. Similarly, Cheung and colleagues[109] found that in a Han Chinese population, HLA-B*15:02 is moderately to strongly predictive of development of severe skin reactions such as Stevens-Johnson syndrome or toxic epidermal necrolysis induced by carbamazepine, phenytoin, or lamotrigine. These are life-threatening complications that appear to occur randomly in clinical settings, so identification of risk alleles can literally be lifesaving. The Clinical Pharmacogenetics Implementation Consortium has proposed guidelines for CYP genotyping to minimize AEs and maximize response for many medication categories including antidepressants[110–112] and antipsychotics.[112]

de Leon[113] suggests that the approach of psychiatric pharmacologic treatment should change: clinicians need to personalize their pharmacologic interventions as much as possible, but the field needs to also consider subdividing psychiatric syndromes into groups that may be more homogeneous for treatment response.

Most current work has focused on single gene variant associations with treatment response or AEs; however, there is some evidence that gene groupings also may be important. For example, although there is no single factor or SNP that is associated with suicidality in major depressive illness, a constellation of genes may predict suicidal activity.[114] Because of the complexity of behavioral symptoms, such gene groupings or gene-gene interactions may be the future of pharmacogenomics in psychiatry.[115]

REFERENCES

1. Winner JG, Carhart JM, Altar CA, et al. A prospective, randomized, double-blind study assessing the clinical impact of integrated pharmacogenomic testing for major depressive disorder. Discov Med 2013;16:219–27.

2. Altar CA, Carhart JM, Allen JD, et al. Clinical validity: combinatorial pharmaco-genomics predicts antidepressant responses and healthcare utilizations better than single gene phenotypes. Pharmacogenomics J 2015;15(5):443–51.

3. Sjöqvist F, Bertilsson L. Clinical pharmacology of antidepressant drugs: phar-macogenetics. Adv Biochem Psychopharmacol 1984;39:359–72.

4. Kane JM, Lieberman J. The efficacy of amoxapine, maprotiline, and trazodone in comparison to imipramine and amitriptyline: a review of the literature. Psycho-pharmacol Bull 1984;20(2):240–9.

5. Burgess CD, Turner P. Cardiotoxicity of antidepressant drugs. Neuropharma-cology 1980;19(12):1195–9.

6. Starkey IR, Lawson AA. Poisoning with tricyclic and related antidepressants–a ten-year review. Q J Med 1980;49(193):33–49.

7. Preskorn SH, Irwin HA. Toxicity of tricyclic antidepressants–kinetics, mecha-nism, intervention: a review. J Clin Psychiatry 1982;43(4):151–6.

8. Chen S, Chou WH, Blouin RA, et al. The cytochrome P450 2D6 (CYP2D6) enzyme polymorphism: screening costs and influence on clinical outcomes in psychiatry. Clin Pharmacol Ther 1996;60(5):522–34.

9. Marshall ZT, Lippmann SB. Tricyclic antidepressant blood levels. Am Fam Physi-cian 1988;37(3):251–4.

10. Schosser A, Serretti A, Souery D, et al. European Group for the Study of Resis-tant Depression (GSRD)–where have we gone so far: review of clinical and ge-netic findings. Eur Neuropsychopharmacol 2012;22(7):453–68.

11. Duan L, Mukherjee EM, Narayan D. Tailoring the treatment of melanoma: impli-cations for personalized medicine. Yale J Biol Med 2015;88(4):389–95.

12. Petric RC, Pop LA, Jurj A, et al. Next generation sequencing applications for breast cancer research. Clujul Med 2015;88(3):278–87.

13. GENDEP Investigators, MARS Investigators, STAR*D Investigators. Common genetic variation and antidepressant efficacy in major depressive disorder: a meta-analysis of three genome-wide pharmacogenetic studies. Am J Psychiatry 2013;170(2):207–17.

14. Winner J, Allen JD, Altar CA, et al. Psychiatric pharmacogenomics predicts health resource utilization of outpatients with anxiety and depression. Transl Psy-chiatry 2013;3:e242.

15. Hall-Flavin DK, Winner JG, Allen JD, et al. Using a pharmacogenomic algorithm to guide the treatment of depression. Transl Psychiatry 2012;2:e172.

16. Rush AJ, Fava M, Wisniewski SR, et al, STAR*D Investigators Group. Sequenced Treatment Alternatives to Relieve Depression (STAR*D): rationale and design. Control Clin Trials 2004;25(1):119–42.

17. Saragoussi D, Chollet J, Bineau S, et al. Antidepressant switching patterns in the treatment of major depressive disorder: a General Practice Research Database (GPRD) study. Int J Clin Pract 2012;66(11):1079–87.

18. Schultz J, Joish V. Costs associated with changes in antidepressant treatment in a managed care population with major depressive disorder. Psychiatr Serv 2009;60(12):1604–11.

19. Warden D, Rush AJ, Wisniewski SR, et al. What predicts attrition in second step medication treatments for depression? A STAR*D Report. Int J Neuropsycho-pharmacol 2009;12(4):459–73.

20. Katz AJ, Dusetzina SB, Farley JF, et al. Distressing adverse events after antide-pressant switch in the Sequenced Treatment Alternatives to Relieve Depression (STAR*D) trial: influence of adverse events during initial treatment with

citalopram on development of subsequent adverse events with an alternative antidepressant. Pharmacotherapy 2012;32(3):234–43.

21. Smits KM, Smits LJ, Schouten JS, et al. Does pretreatment testing for serotonin transporter polymorphisms lead to earlier effects of drug treatment in patients with major depression? A decision-analytic model. Clin Ther 2007;29(4): 691–702.

22. Serretti A, Olgiati P, Bajo E, et al. A model to incorporate genetic testing (5-HTTLPR) in pharmacological treatment of major depressive disorders. World J Biol Psychiatry 2011;12(7):501–15.

23. Hornberger J, Li Q, Quinn B. Cost-effectiveness of combinatorial pharmacogenomic testing for treatment-resistant major depressive disorder patients. Am J Manag Care 2015;21(6):e357–65.

24. Lanktree MB, Zai G, Vanderbeek LE, et al. Positive perception of pharmacogenetic testing for psychotropic medications. Hum Psychopharmacol 2014;29(3): 287–91.

25. Thomas JH. Rapid birth–death evolution specific to xenobiotic cytochrome P450 genes in vertebrates. PLoS Genet 2007;3(5):e67.

26. Zanger UM, Schwab M. Cytochrome P450 enzymes in drug metabolism: regulation of gene expression, enzyme activities, and impact of genetic variation. Pharmacol Ther 2013;138(1):103–41.

27. Polimanti R, Piacentini S, Manfellotto D, et al. Human genetic variation of CYP450 superfamily. Pharmacogenomics 2012;13(16):1951–60.

28. Chen Q, Zhang T, Wang JF, et al. Advances in human cytochrome p450 and personalized medicine. Curr Drug Metab 2011;12(5):436–44.

29. Eap CB, Bender S, Sirot EJ, et al. Nonresponse to clozapine and ultrarapid CYP1A2 activity: clinical data and analysis of CYP1A2 gene. J Clin Psychopharmacol 2004;24(2):214–9.

30. Narahari A, El-Mallakh RS, Kolikonda MK, et al. How coffee and cigarettes can effect the response to psychopharmacotherapy. Current Psychiatry 2015; 14(10):79–80.

31. Xu Q, Wu X, Li M, et al. Association studies of genomic variants with treatment response to risperidone, clozapine, quetiapine and chlorpromazine in the Chinese Han population. Pharmacogenomics J 2015. [Epub ahead of print].

32. van de Bilt MT, Prado CM, Ojopi EP, et al. Cytochrome P450 genotypes are not associated with refractoriness to antipsychotic treatment. Schizophr Res 2015; 168(1–2):587–8.

33. Lanni C, Racchi M, Govoni S. Do we need pharmacogenetics to personalize antidepressant therapy? Cell Mol Life Sci 2013;70(18):3327–40.

34. Caspi A, Sugden K, Moffitt TE, et al. Influence of life stress on depression: moderation by a polymorphism in the 5-HTT gene. Science 2003;301:386–9.

35. Luddington NA, Mandadapu A, Husk M, et al. Clinical implications of genetic variation in the serotonin transporter promoter region: a review. Prim Care Companion J Clin Psychiatry 2009;11(3):93–102.

36. Karlović D, Karlović D. Serotonin transporter gene (5-HTTLPR) polymorphism and efficacy of selective serotonin reuptake inhibitors–do we have sufficient evidence for clinical practice. Acta Clin Croat 2013;52(3):353–62.

37. Heils A, Teufel A, Petri S, et al. Allelic variation of human serotonin transporter gene expression. J Neurochem 1996;66(6):2621–4.

38. Bradley SL, Dodelzon K, Sandhu HK, et al. Relationship of serotonin transporter gene polymorphisms and haplotypes to mRNA transcription. Am J Med Genet B Neuropsychiatr Genet 2005;136(1):58–61.

39. Kaiser R, Müller-Oerlinghausen B, Filler D, et al. Correlation between serotonin uptake in human blood platelets with the 44-bp polymorphism and the 17-bp variable number tandem repeat of the serotonin transporter. Am J Med Genet 2002;114(3):323–8.
40. Serretti A, Olgiati P, Liebman MN, et al. Clinical prediction of antidepressant response in mood disorders: linear multivariate vs. neural network models. Psychiatry Res 2007;152(2–3):223–31.
41. Kato M, Serretti A. Review and meta-analysis of antidepressant pharmacogenetic findings in major depressive disorder. Mol Psychiatry 2010;15(5):473–500.
42. El-Mallakh RS, Gao Y, Briscoe BT, et al. Tardive dysphoria: the role of long term antidepressant use in inducing chronic depression. Med Hypotheses 2011; 80(1):57–9.
43. Parsey RV, Hastings RS, Oquendo MA, et al. Effect of a triallelic functional polymorphism of the serotonin-transporter-linked promoter region on expression of serotonin transporter in the human brain. Am J Psychiatry 2006;163(1):48–51.
44. Benedetti F, Dallaspezia S, Colombo C, et al. Effect of catechol-O-methyltransferase Val(108/158)Met polymorphism on antidepressant efficacy of fluvoxamine. Eur Psychiatry 2010;25(8):476–8.
45. Hopkins SC, Reasner DS, Koblan KS. Catechol-O-methyltransferase genotype as modifier of superior responses to venlafaxine treatment in major depressive disorder. Psychiatry Res 2013;208(3):285–7.
46. Atake K, Yoshimura R, Hori H, et al. Catechol-O-methyltransferase Val158Met genotype and the clinical responses to duloxetine treatment or plasma levels of 3-methoxy-4-hydroxyphenylglycol and homovanillic acid in Japanese patients with major depressive disorder. Neuropsychiatr Dis Treat 2015;11:967–74.
47. Lin JY, Jiang MY, Kan ZM, et al. Influence of 5-HTR2A genetic polymorphisms on the efficacy of antidepressants in the treatment of major depressive disorder: a meta-analysis. J Affect Disord 2014;168:430–8.
48. Kautzky A, Baldinger P, Souery D, et al. The combined effect of genetic polymorphisms and clinical parameters on treatment outcome in treatment-resistant depression. Eur Neuropsychopharmacol 2015;25(4):441–53.
49. Villafuerte SM, Vallabhaneni K, Sliwerska E, et al. SSRI response in depression may be influenced by SNPs in HTR1B and HTR1A. Psychiatr Genet 2009;19(6): 281–91.
50. Nase S, Köhler S, Jennebach J, et al. Role of serum brain derived neurotrophic factor and central N-Acetylaspartate for clinical response under antidepressive pharmacotherapy. Neurosignals 2016;24(1):1–14.
51. Kocabas NA, Antonijevic I, Faghel C, et al. Brain-derived neurotrophic factor gene polymorphisms: influence on treatment response phenotypes of major depressive disorder. Int Clin Psychopharmacol 2011;26(1):1–10.
52. Su N, Zhang L, Fei F, et al. The brain-derived neurotrophic factor is associated with alcohol dependence-related depression and antidepressant response. Brain Res 2011;1415:119–26.
53. Musil R, Zill P, Seemüller F, et al. No influence of brain-derived neurotrophic factor (BDNF) polymorphisms on treatment response in a naturalistic sample of patients with major depression. Eur Arch Psychiatry Clin Neurosci 2013;263(5): 405–12.
54. Perlis RH, Moorjani P, Fagerness J, et al. Pharmacogenetic analysis of genes implicated in rodent models of antidepressant response: association of TREK1 and treatment resistance in the STAR*D Study. Neuropsychopharmacology 2008;33:2810–9.

55. Heurteaux C, Lucas G, Guy N, et al. Deletion of the background potassium channel TREK-1 results in a depression-resistant phenotype. Nat Neurosci 2006;9:1134–41.

56. Huang X, Yu T, Li X, et al. *ABCB6, ABCB1* and *ABCG1* genetic polymorphisms and antidepressant response of SSRIs in Chinese depressive patients. Pharmacogenomics 2013;14(14):1723–30.

57. Breitenstein B, Brückl TM, Ising M, et al. *ABCB1* gene variants and antidepressant treatment outcome: a meta-analysis. Am J Med Genet B Neuropsychiatr Genet 2015;168B(4):274–83.

58. Breitenstein B, Scheuer S, Brückl TM, et al. Association of ABCB1 gene variants, plasma antidepressant concentration, and treatment response: results from a randomized clinical study. J Psychiatr Res 2015;73:86–95.

59. Chang HH, Chou CH, Yang YK, et al. Association between ABCB1 polymorphisms and antidepressant treatment response in Taiwanese major depressive patients. Clin Psychopharmacol Neurosci 2015;13(3):250–5.

60. Ray A, Tennakoon L, Keller J, et al. *ABCB1* (MDR1) predicts remission on P-gp substrates in chronic depression. Pharmacogenomics J 2015;15(4):332–9.

61. Breitenstein B, Scheuer S, Pfister H, et al. The clinical application of ABCB1 genotyping in antidepressant treatment: a pilot study. CNS Spectr 2014;19(2): 165–75.

62. Kirchheiner J, Lorch R, Lebedeva E, et al. Genetic variants in FKBP5 affecting response to antidepressant drug treatment. Pharmacogenomics 2008;9(7): 841–6.

63. Stamm TJ, Rampp C, Wiethoff K, et al. The *FKBP5* polymorphism rs1360780 influences the effect of an algorithm-based antidepressant treatment and is associated with remission in patients with major depression. J Psychopharmacol 2016;30(1):40–7.

64. Hu Q, Zhang SY, Liu F, et al. Influence of *GNB3* C825T polymorphism on the efficacy of antidepressants in the treatment of major depressive disorder: a meta-analysis. J Affect Disord 2014;172C:103–9.

65. Fabbri C, Marsano A, Albani D, et al. *PPP3CC* gene: a putative modulator of antidepressant response through the B-cell receptor signaling pathway. Pharmacogenomics J 2014;14(5):463–72.

66. Jiang W, Xu J, Lu XJ, et al. Association between *MTHFR* C677T polymorphism and depression: a meta-analysis in the Chinese population. Psychol Health Med 2015. [Epub ahead of print].

67. Papakostas GI, Shelton RC, Zajecka JM, et al. L-methylfolate as adjunctive therapy for SSRI-resistant major depression: results of two randomized, double-blind, parallel-sequential trials. Am J Psychiatry 2012;169(12):1267–74.

68. Papakostas GI, Shelton RC, Zajecka JM, et al. Effect of adjunctive L-methylfolate 15 mg among inadequate responders to SSRIs in depressed patients who were stratified by biomarker levels and genotype: results from a randomized clinical trial. J Clin Psychiatry 2014;75(8):855–63.

69. Mischoulon D, Lamon-Fava S, Selhub J, et al. Prevalence of *MTHFR* C677T and MS A2756G polymorphisms in major depressive disorder, and their impact on response to fluoxetine treatment. CNS Spectr 2012;17(2):76–86.

70. Schizophrenia Working Group of the Psychiatric Genomics Consortium. Biological insights from 108 schizophrenia-associated genetic loci. Nature 2014;511: 421–7.

71. Lencz T, Robinson DG, Xu K, et al. *DRD2* promoter region variation as a predictor of sustained response to antipsychotic medication in first-episode schizophrenia patients. Am J Psychiatry 2006;163:529–31.

72. Zhang JP, Lencz T, Malhotra AK. D2 receptor genetic variation and clinical response to antipsychotic drug treatment: a meta-analysis. Am J Psychiatry 2010;167:763–72.

73. Zhang JP, Robinson DG, Gallego JA, et al. Association of a schizophrenia risk variant at the DRD2 locus with antipsychotic treatment response in first-episode psychosis. Schizophr Bull 2015;41(6):1248–55.

74. Kang SG, Na KS, Lee HJ, et al. *DRD2* genotypic and haplotype variation is associated with improvements in negative symptoms after 6 weeks' amisulpride treatment. J Clin Psychopharmacol 2015;35(2):158–62.

75. Lewis AG, Minchin RF. Lack of exonic sulfotransferase 4A1 mutations in controls and schizophrenia cases. Psychiatr Genet 2009;19(1):53–5.

76. Meltzer HY, Brennan MD, Woodward ND, et al. Association of *Sult4A1* SNPs with psychopathology and cognition in patients with schizophrenia or schizoaffective disorder. Schizophr Res 2008;106(2–3):258–64.

77. Ramsey TL, Meltzer HY, Brock GN, et al. Evidence for a *SULT4A1* haplotype correlating with baseline psychopathology and atypical antipsychotic response. Pharmacogenomics 2011;12(4):471–80.

78. Liu Q, Ramsey TL, Meltzer HY, et al. Sulfotransferase 4A1 haplotype 1 (*SULT4A1-1*) is associated with decreased hospitalization events in antipsychotic-treated patients with schizophrenia. Pharmacogenomics 2011; 12(4):471–80.

79. Wang D, Li Q, Favis R, et al. *SULT4A1* haplotype: conflicting results on its role as a biomarker of antipsychotic response. Pharmacogenomics 2014;15(12): 1557–64.

80. Huo R, Wei Z, Xiong Y, et al. Association of dopamine receptor D1 (*DRD1*) polymorphisms with risperidone treatment response in Chinese schizophrenia patients. Neurosci Lett 2015;584:178–83.

81. de Matos LP, Santana CV, Souza RP. Meta-analysis of dopamine receptor D1 rs4532 polymorphism and susceptibility to antipsychotic treatment response. Psychiatry Res 2015;229(1–2):586–8.

82. Souza RP, Meltzer HY, Lieberman JA, et al. Influence of neurexin 1 (*NRXN1*) polymorphisms in clozapine response. Hum Psychopharmacol 2010;25(7–8): 582–5.

83. Jenkins A, Apud JA, Zhang F, et al. Identification of candidate single-nucleotide polymorphisms in *NRXN1* related to antipsychotic treatment response in patients with schizophrenia. Neuropsychopharmacology 2014;39(9):2170–8.

84. Terzić T, Kastelic M, Dolžan V, et al. Influence of 5-HT1A and 5-HTTLPR genetic variants on the schizophrenia symptoms and occurrence of treatment-resistant schizophrenia. Neuropsychiatr Dis Treat 2015;11:453–9.

85. Fonseka TM, Tiwari AK, Gonçalves VF, et al. The role of genetic variation across IL-1β, IL-2, IL-6, and BDNF in antipsychotic-induced weight gain. World J Biol Psychiatry 2015;16(1):45–56.

86. Bosia M, Lorenzi C, Pirovano A, et al. *COMT* Val158Met and 5-HT1A-R -1019 C/ G polymorphisms: effects on the negative symptom response to clozapine. Pharmacogenomics 2015;16(1):35–44.

87. Grove T, Taylor S, Dalack G, et al. Endothelial function, folate pharmacogenomics, and neurocognition in psychotic disorders. Schizophr Res 2015;164(1–3): 115–21.

88. Tiwari AK, Brandl EJ, Zai CC, et al. Association of orexin receptor polymorphisms with antipsychotic-induced weight gain. World J Biol Psychiatry 2016; 17(3):221–9.
89. Shi S, Leites C, He D, et al. MicroRNA-9 and microRNA-326 regulate human dopamine D2 receptor expression, and the microRNA-mediated expression regulation is altered by a genetic variant. J Biol Chem 2014;289(19):13434–44.
90. Kao AC, Rojnic Kuzman M, Tiwari AK, et al. Methylenetetrahydrofolate reductase gene variants and antipsychotic-induced weight gain and metabolic disturbances. J Psychiatr Res 2014;54:36–42.
91. Roffeei SN, Reynolds GP, Zainal NZ, et al. Association of ADRA2A and MTHFR gene polymorphisms with weight loss following antipsychotic switching to aripiprazole or ziprasidone. Hum Psychopharmacol 2014;29(1):38–45.
92. Roffeei SN, Mohamed Z, Reynolds GP, et al. Association of FTO, LEPR and MTHFR gene polymorphisms with metabolic syndrome in schizophrenia patients receiving antipsychotics. Pharmacogenomics 2014;15(4):477–85.
93. Wang F, Mi W, Ma W, et al. A pharmacogenomic study revealed an association between SLC6A4 and risperidone-induced weight gain in Chinese Han population. Pharmacogenomics 2015;16(17):1943–9.
94. Lovallo WR, King AC, Farag NH, et al. Naltrexone effects on cortisol secretion in women and men in relation to a family history of alcoholism: studies from the Oklahoma family health patterns project. Psychoneuroendocrinology 2012; 37(12):1922–8.
95. Krystal JH, Cramer JA, Krol WF, et al, Veterans Affairs Naltrexone Cooperative Study 425 Group. Naltrexone in the treatment of alcohol dependence. N Engl J Med 2001;345:1734–9.
96. Gastpar M, Bonnet U, Böning J, et al. Lack of efficacy of naltrexone in the prevention of alcohol relapse: results from a German multicenter study. J Clin Psychopharmacol 2002;22(6):592–8.
97. Oslin DW, Berrettini W, Kranzler HR, et al. A functional polymorphism of the mu-opioid receptor gene is associated with naltrexone response in alcohol-dependent patients. Neuropsychopharmacology 2003;28(8):1546–52.
98. Ray LA, Bujarski S, Chin PF, et al. Pharmacogenetics of naltrexone in Asian Americans: a randomized placebo-controlled laboratory study. Neuropsychopharmacology 2012;37:445–55.
99. Gelernter J, Gueorguieva R, Kranzler HR, et al, VA Cooperative Study #425 Study Group. Opioid receptor gene (OPRM1, OPRK1, and OPRD1) variants and response to naltrexone treatment for alcohol dependence: results from the VA Cooperative Study. Alcohol Clin Exp Res 2007;31(4):555–63.
100. Karpyak VM, Biernacka JM, Geske JR, et al. Genetic markers associated with abstinence length in alcohol-dependent subjects treated with acamprosate. Translational Psychiatry 2014;4:e453.
101. Spellicy CJ, Kosten TR, Hamon SC, et al. The MTHFR C677T variant is associated with responsiveness to disulfiram treatment for cocaine dependency. Front Psychiatry 2012;3:109.
102. CDC Center for Public Health. Genomics, U.S. genome variation estimates: MTHFR allele and genotype frequencies. Available at: http://www.cdc.gov/genomics/population/file/print/genvar/mthfr.pdf. Accessed January 20, 2016.
103. NIH NCBI Bookshelf. Chapter 3, pharmacology of medications used to treat opioid addiction. 2005. Available at: http://www.ncbi.nim.nih.gov. Accessed January 12, 2016.

104. Bart G, Kreek MJ, Ott J, et al. Increased attributable risk related to a functional mu-opioid receptor gene polymorphism in association with alcohol dependence in central Sweden. Neuropsychopharmacology 2005;30(2):417–22.

105. Reynolds KK, Ramey Hartung B, Jortani SA. The value of CYP2D6 and OPRM1 pharmacogenetic testing for opioid therapy. Clin Lab Med 2008;28:581–98.

106. Crist RC, Clarke TM, Ang A, et al. An intronic variant in OPRD1 predicts treatment outcome for opioid dependence in African-Americans. Neuropsychopharmacology 2013;38:2003–10.

107. Clarke TK, Crist RC, Ang A, et al. Genetic variation in OPRD1 and the response to treatment for opioid dependence with buprenorphine in European-American females. Pharmacogenomics J 2014;14(3):303–8.

108. Verbelen M, Lewis CM. How close are we to a pharmacogenomic test for clozapine-induced agranulocytosis? Pharmacogenomics 2015;16(9):915–7.

109. Cheung YK, Cheng SH, Chan EJ, et al. HLA-B alleles associated with severe cutaneous reactions to antiepileptic drugs in Han Chinese. Epilepsia 2013; 54(7):1307–14.

110. Hicks JK, Swen JJ, Thorn CF, et al, Clinical Pharmacogenetics Implementation Consortium. Clinical pharmacogenetics implementation consortium guideline for CYP2D6 and CYP2C19 genotypes and dosing of tricyclic antidepressants. Clin Pharmacol Ther 2013;93(5):402–8.

111. Hicks JK, Bishop JR, Sangkuhl K, et al, Clinical Pharmacogenetics Implementation Consortium. Clinical pharmacogenetics implementation consortium (CPIC) guideline for CYP2D6 and CYP2C19 genotypes and dosing of selective serotonin reuptake inhibitors. Clin Pharmacol Ther 2015;98(2):127–34.

112. Swen JJ, Nijenhuis M, de Boer A, et al. Pharmacogenetics: from bench to byte– an update of guidelines. Clin Pharmacol Ther 2011;89(5):662–73.

113. de Leon J. Focusing on drug versus disease mechanisms and on clinical subgrouping to advance personalised medicine in psychiatry. Acta Neuropsychiatr 2014;26(6):327–33.

114. Mullins N, Perroud N, Uher R, et al. Genetic relationships between suicide attempts, suicidal ideation and major psychiatric disorders: a genome-wide association and polygenic scoring study. Am J Med Genet B Neuropsychiatr Genet 2014;165B(5):428–37.

115. Lim CH, Zain SM, Reynolds GP, et al. Genetic association of LMAN2L gene in schizophrenia and bipolar disorder and its interaction with ANK3 gene polymorphism. Prog Neuropsychopharmacol Biol Psychiatry 2014;54:157–62.

Clinical Utility and Economic Impact of CYP2D6 Genotyping

 CrossMark

Kristen K. Reynolds, PhD[a,b,*], Beth A. McNally, PhD[a],
Mark W. Linder, PhD, DABCC[a,b]

KEYWORDS

- CYP2D6 • CYP2D6 genotyping • Pharmacogenetics • Pharmacoeconomics

KEY POINTS

- Correlation of genotyping with clinical outcomes and cost.
- CYP2D6 genotyping can affect efficacy, toxicity, and costs associated with psychiatric, pain, and cardiovascular medications.
- The development of pharmacogenetics guidelines provide improved understanding and application of genotyping results in practice.

INTRODUCTION

Considerable progress has been made in pharmacogenetics over the past decade, resulting in increased awareness and availability of pharmacogenetic diagnostics in the clinical setting. Currently, more than 130 drugs are approved by the US Food and Drug Administration (FDA) that contain pharmacogenetic information in the package label inserts.[1] Initiatives such as the Clinical Pharmacogenetics Implementation Consortium (CPIC) have been developed to generate up-to-date guidelines based on systematic review of the vastly increasing literature base to assist physicians and pharmacists with pharmacogenetic-based dosing strategies.[2,3]

Undoubtedly, pharmacogenetic testing of the cytochrome P450 2D6 (CYP2D6) has been at the forefront of personalized medicine. CYP2D6 genotyping has been extremely valuable in identifying individuals likely to have altered reactions to various pharmaceuticals and for predicting patient response. The protein product encoded by the CYP2D6 gene is classified as a monooxygenase and is responsible for metabolizing roughly 25% of all commonly prescribed drugs, including opioids,

[a] PGXL Laboratories, 201 East Jefferson Street, Suite 309, Louisville, KY 40202, USA;
[b] Department of Pathology and Laboratory Medicine, University of Louisville School of Medicine, 323 East Chestnut Street, Louisville, KY 40292, USA
* Corresponding author. PGXL Laboratories, 201 East Jefferson Street, Suite 309, Louisville, KY 40202.
E-mail address: kreynolds@pgxlab.com

Clin Lab Med 36 (2016) 525–542
http://dx.doi.org/10.1016/j.cll.2016.05.008
0272-2712/16/$ – see front matter © 2016 Elsevier Inc. All rights reserved.
labmed.theclinics.com

many antidepressants, antipsychotics, beta-blockers, and tamoxifen.[4–7] The highly polymorphic CYP2D6 gene is subject to copy number variations, single-nucleotide polymorphisms and additional genetic modifications, such as insertions and deletions, each of which may alter individual responses to medications via changes in drug metabolism. Thus far, the Cytochrome P450 Nomenclature Committee (http://www.cypalleles.ki.se) has catalogued and recognized more than 100 CYP2D6 alleles, and many laboratories certified by Clinical Laboratory Improvement Amendments (CLIA) offer targeted variant analysis of the CYP2D6 gene.[8] Detecting variants of the CYP2D6 gene that alter CYP2D6 enzymatic activity can identify patients with increased risk of adverse drug reactions (ADRs) or therapeutic failure to standard dosages of medications metabolized by CYP2D6.

A clinically valuable result from CYP2D6 genotyping is identification of the CYP2D6 poor metabolizer (PM) phenotype. In some individuals, the CYP2D6 gene is completely absent, whereas other individuals carry 2 variant alleles that encode nonfunctional enzymes. In this instance, the genotype dictates the phenotype, which is not subject to external influences such as the effect of CYP2D6 inhibitors or environmentally induced epigenetic changes. Although ethnic background can vary the distribution, approximately 7% to 10% of the general population is genetic CYP2D6 PMs with no CYP2D6 enzymatic activity.[9] In this scenario, reduced metabolic clearance rates result in accumulation of drug concentrations above the therapeutic range. Thus, in PMs, standard dosage rates significantly exceed the standard dosage rate, which increases side-effect risk. Another 10% to 50% of the population (depending on ethnicity) is considered intermediate metabolizers (IMs).[7] Individuals with the CYP2D6 IM phenotype inherit 1 inactive allele that codes for a loss of function enzyme or 2 alleles that encode enzymes with decreased activity.[7] Although some recent studies suggest that individuals who carry 1 inactive allele and 1 active or wild type allele (eg, CYP2D6*1/*4) could be classified as extensive metabolizers (EMs) based on CYP2D6 activity scores.[10] The CPIC has just recently finalized a standardization for phenotype designations that defines that allele combination as IM based on decreased overall metabolic clearance.[11] Both IMs and PMs, approximately 45% of the white and African American populations, exhibit decreased metabolic activity and an increased risk for side effects to drugs normally inactivated by CYP2D6 (eg, amitriptyline, metoprolol), or lack of efficacy for drugs requiring activation by CYP2D6 (eg, prodrugs such as codeine, oxycodone, tamoxifen). Another 1% to 6% of the general population constitutes CYP2D6 ultrarapid metabolizers (UMs).[12] Individuals identified with the UM phenotype have 3 or more wild type copies of the CYP2D6 gene and, at the other extreme, have higher than normal enzymatic activity. UMs are at increased risk of failure for active drugs because they clear the drugs too rapidly to benefit from a standard dose by not allowing the drug to reach minimum therapeutic concentrations. UMs are also at increased risk of toxic side effects from prodrugs because they convert the drug into an active form more so than expected, resulting in an excess dose of the drug's active metabolite.[13,14]

The association of CYP2D6 genotype to phenotype is best detailed by focusing on specific drugs and/or drug classes. There is a significant association of the PM phenotype to decreased metabolic clearance and increased risk of ADRs in patients treated with tricyclic antidepressants (TCAs), antipsychotics, opioids, and antiarrhythmic medications. For example, knowing the patient's CYP2D6 genotype allows the physician to identify PM patients at risk for ADRs and either significantly lower dosage rates to account for decreased metabolic clearance rate or avoid prescribing the drug altogether. Additionally, knowledge of the CYP2D6 genotype can allow physicians to identify patients at risk of therapeutic failure given their inability to acti-vate prodrugs and instead consider alternative medications to increase the likelihood of an efficacious response, and decrease a prescription process based on trial and error.

CLINICAL UTILITY: 2D6 STRONG GENE-DRUG CORRELATIONS

A significant body of clinical evidence exists to support actionable, quantitative dose adjustments for certain drugs in individuals with CYP2D6 genetic variants. The Dutch Pharmacogenetics Working Group (DPWG) has reviewed more than 500 references published in the last 2 decades that demonstrate an association of phenotype to drug safety and efficacy.[14] The objective of the DPWG is to develop pharmacogenetic-based therapeutic dose recommendations based on a systematic review of the literature with the goal of assisting clinicians, pharmacists, and other practitioners with a working integration of genotyping data for therapeutic guidance. The results of their review and those of the CPIC (www.pharmgkb.org) are summa-rized in **Table 1**.

A brief description of how the recommendations were concluded is important because the data are directly calculated from peer-reviewed literature. Level of evidence for the gene-drug interaction was scored on a 5-point scale in which a higher numbered rating denotes those studies demonstrating a strong correlation of pheno-type to clinical outcome. The classification of clinical relevance was scored on a 7-point lettered scale derived from the National Cancer Institute's Common Toxicity Criteria, wherein a clinical effect that was not significant was scored AA, whereas an event such as an arrhythmia or death was scored F (see **Table 1**). In addition to the scoring criteria, calculated dose adjustments to correct blood concentrations to norms for patients with extensive metabolism was based on 4 rules: (1) pharmaco-kinetic data were only used from papers that scored 3 or 4; (2) only statistically significant data were used to calculate doses; (3) for active drugs, calculations were based on the sum of parent drug and active metabolites; and (4) for prodrugs, the pharmacokinetics of the active metabolite were used. In this manner, the bias towards increased risk of concentration-dependent adverse events for PMs, IMs, and UMs was minimized.

This article addresses the utility of pharmacogenetic testing for cross-disciplinary medications metabolized through the CYP2D6 pathway. It provides a compilation of the most clinically pressing applications of CYP2D6 genotyping and an update of the current clinical impact of CYP2D6 genetic testing, focusing on evidence-based rationale for clinical relevance and cost-effectiveness because strength of clinical evidence and endorsement by professional guidelines have been cited as 2 of the most significant factors influencing reimbursement.[15,16] This article draws examples from psychology, cardiology, and pain management medications because these specialties have, thus far, gained the most from pharmacogenetic testing.

PSYCHIATRY

Several psychotropic medications are metabolized by CYP2D6. The efficacy of many antipsychotics and antidepressants, including selective serotonin reuptake inhibitors (SSRIs), nonselective reuptake inhibitors, and TCAs, are influenced by CYP2D6 meta-bolic function. Notably, CYP2D6 PM phenotype is linked to increased risk of toxicity for several psychotropics, such as paroxetine,[17] fluvoxamine,[17] amitriptyline, desipra-mine, haloperidol, risperidone, and venlafaxine (VEN).[18–21] A substantial evidence

Table 1
Body of evidence for CYP2D6 clinical implications

Drug	PM Score	Action for PM	UM Score	Action for UM
Amitriptyline	3A	50% decrease (or avoid)	3C	Avoid
Clomipramine	4C	50% decrease (or avoid)	2C	Avoid
Doxepin	3F	50%–60% decrease (or avoid)	3A	Avoid or 100% increase
Imipramine	4C	50%–70% decrease (or avoid)	4C	Avoid or 70% increase
Nortriptyline	3C	50%–60% decrease (or avoid)	3C	Avoid or 60% increase
Venlafaxine	4C	Avoid	4A	Avoid or 150% increase
Aripiprazole	4C	33%–50% decrease	—	—
Haloperidol	4C	50% decrease (or avoid)	4C	Avoid or adjust to [plasma]
Risperidone	4D	Avoid	4C	Avoid
Codeine	4B	Avoid or be alert to failure	3F	Avoid or be alert to ADR
Oxycodone	3B	Avoid or be alert to failure	1A	Avoid or be alert to ADR
Metoprolol	4C	Avoid or 75% decrease	4D	Avoid or 250% increase
Propafenone	4C	70% decrease	3D	Avoid or adjust to EKG and [plasma]
Tamoxifen	4E	Avoid	4A	—

[a] Level of evidence: Quality of evidence for gene–drug interaction is 0, lowest evidence; 4, highest evidence.
[b] Clinical relevance of gene–drug interaction: AA, lowest impact; F, highest impact.
Data from Swen JJ, Nijenhuis M, De Boer A, et al. Pharmacogenetics: from bench to byte—an update of guidelines. Clin Pharmacol Ther 2011;89(5):662–73; and Hicks JK, Swen JJ, Thorn CF, et al. Clinical Pharmacogenetics Implementation Consortium guideline for CYP2D6 and CYP2C19 genotypes and dosing of tricyclic antidepressants. Clin Pharmacol Ther 2013;93(5):402–8.

base exists that correlates therapeutic inefficacy of antidepressants with the CYP2D6 UM phenotype.[14,17] In general, CYP2D6 PMs are at risk of toxicity due to decreased elimination and increased half-life of a CYP2D6-dependent drug in the blood, whereas CYP2D6 UMs may require increased dose requirements due to increased metabolism or elimination of a given drug.

Tricyclic Antidepressants: Amitriptyline, Clomipramine, Doxepin, Imipramine, and Nortriptyline

CYP2D6 deficiencies result in significantly elevated plasma concentrations of TCAs, ranging from 2 to 80 times the therapeutic concentrations.[22] Supratherapeutic drug levels increase the risk of side effects, including anticholinergic effects (eg, blurred vision, dizziness), cardiotoxic effects (eg, arrhythmia, orthostatic hypotension), and central nervous system toxicities (eg, seizures, delirium). In the CPIC guideline for TCAs, Hicks and colleagues[8] demonstrated that a clear correlation exists between CYP2D6 genotype and adverse event risk in patients treated with TCAs. Both amitriptyline and nortriptyline were used as model drugs for the CPIC guidelines because most pharmacogenomics studies have focused on these 2 drugs. However, the review indicates that other tricyclics have comparable pharmacokinetic properties and adverse event profiles. For CYP2D6 PMs, the CPIC guidelines indicate avoidance of amitriptyline and a dose reduction of 50% to 70% for clomipramine, doxepin, nortriptyline, and imipramine (see **Table 1**). Practical application of this information to determine dosing can eliminate risk bias introduced by attenuated clearance capacity of individual patients and thus improve clinical outcomes and decrease the failure rate of antidepressant therapy.

Systematic review and strength of data scoring provided by the CPIC and DPWG, also indicate that CYP2D6 genotyping is sufficiently supported for patients being treated with certain other antidepressants, antipsychotics, opioids, and cardiovascular drugs such as VEN, risperidone, haloperidol, aripiprazole, codeine, and metoprolol.

Venlafaxine

VEN is a mixed serotonin and norepinephrine reuptake inhibitor commonly used as first-line treatment of depression. It is metabolized by CYP2D6 to a metabolite o-desmethylvenlafaxine (ODV) that is equally as active as the parent compound (VEN). Studies have demonstrated that CYP2D6 PMs taking VEN do not produce appreciable levels of the ODV metabolite, and demonstrate plasma ODV to VEN ratios that are 6 times lower than the mean of the total tested cohort containing all genotypes.[18] Compared with normal metabolizers, PM patients experience up to 4 times more adverse events, including nausea, vomiting, and diarrhea.[18–20] Additionally, there have been case studies reporting severe arrhythmias in 4 subjects treated with VEN who all were CYP2D6 PMs.[21] In another study, 5 subjects with the IM phenotype (who lack a fully active CYP2D6 allele) could not tolerate VEN doses above 75 mg per day and all except 1 discontinued the VEN treatment because of intolerable side effects.[20]

On systematic review of the VEN literature, the DPWG determined that a population size-weighted mean dose adjustment could not be determined for CYP2D6 PM patients.[14] It was not possible to calculate a dose reduction that both reduced the risk for side effects but also retained efficacy because the therapeutic efficacy, not the side effects, relate to the sum of VEN and ODV plasma concentrations. For this reason, the DPWG recommends that VEN be avoided in PM patients (see **Table 1**).

Antipsychotropic Medications: Risperidone, Haloperidol, and Aripiprazole

Risperidone

Risperidone is an atypical antipsychotic medication used to treat schizophrenia, bipolar disorder, and psychotic depression. Risperidone is among the most commonly prescribed antipsychotic medications in the United States. Dose-dependent symptoms include drowsiness, sedation, tachycardia, hypotension, extrapyramidal symptoms (EPS), tardive dyskinesia (which can be permanent), and, rarely, the potentially fatal neuroleptic-malignant syndrome (NMS).[23,24]

Several studies and case reports in the last decade have consistently demonstrated a significantly increased risk of ADRs in CYP2D6 PM subjects taking risperidone.[25-30] The DPWG determined by systematic review that the level of evidence for the clinical 2D6-risperidone interaction was strong enough to suggest that 2D6 PMs avoid risperidone (see **Table 1**).

De Leon and colleagues[26] showed that CYP2D6 genotype is significantly associated with risperidone ADR risk. This study demonstrated that CYP2D6 PM subjects taking risperidone exhibit (1) higher plasma concentrations of risperidone, (2) a 3.4-fold increased risk of experiencing a moderate to severe risperidone ADR, and (3) a 6-fold increased risk of discontinuing therapy due to risperidone ADRs. In this study, the CYP2D6 PM phenotype was the only significant variable in multivariate logistic regression models to correlate with risk of risperidone ADR and discontinuation. Considering that the relapse rate in schizophrenic patients ranges from 19% to 100%,[31] and hospitalization for relapse increases cost by 5-fold[32] (**Table 5**), a 6-fold increased risk of discontinuing risperidone due to ADRs represents a significant risk to relapse rate, hospitalization risk, and cost burden.

Haloperidol

Haloperidol is a common antipsychotic used to treat schizophrenia; however, the drug comes with a high incidence of ADR risk of serious EPS, including dystonia, pseudoparkinsonism, akathisia, and tardive dyskinesia, as well as leukopenia and arrhythmias.[23] Brockmoller and colleagues[33] showed that, compared with CYP2D6 normal metabolizers, CYP2D6 PMs have statistically significant decreases in plasma haloperidol clearance rates, increased plasma haloperidol metabolite concentrations, and a corresponding statistically significant 2-fold higher EPS rate. In this study, 80% of the CYP2D6 PMs experienced significant EPS.

After review of the published plasma concentration differences and EPS rates among CYP2D6 PMs, the DPWG calculated a scientific evidence score that warrants a haloperidol dose reduction of 50% for PMs.[14] The 50% dose reduction recommendation takes into consideration the decreased drug clearance experienced by CYP2D6 PMs and ultimately serves to normalize EPS risk. An understanding that the mechanism of risk of haloperidol use is due to decreased clearance in CYP2D6 PMs allows the physician to take action based on the metabolic mechanism and decrease the standard haloperidol dose in these patients by 50%. Thus, it is the CYP2D6 genotype that provides the critical piece of information necessary to account for the defect in clearance so that the dose can be adjusted accordingly before an adverse event occurs.

Aripiprazole

In 2013, Abilify (aripiprazole) was the best-selling prescription drug in the United States.[34] Dose-related adverse reactions include somnolence, tremor, EPS, and akasthisia.[35] CYP2D6 PMs have increased drug exposure and an increased risk of developing these dose-related ADRs. In a small case-controlled study, the authors found an association of CYP2D6 deficient genotypes in adolescents who developed EPS, 1 of whom developed an NMS-like reaction.[36] The study demonstrated that children with CYP2D6 abnormalities were at increased risk of aripiprazole-induced ADRs. These dose-dependent adverse events are significant and, in the case of some EPS, can be permanent.

Systematic review of literature regarding CYP2D6 genotyping for aripiprazole treatment by the DPWG revealed that adverse events significantly correlated with CYP2D6 phenotype.[37] The DPWG calculated that the population size-weighted mean of the dose adjustment was 63% to 68% of the normal recommended dose. For clinical applicability, this translates to a dose reduction of 33%, or 67% of the recommended maximum, which is equivalent to a maximum daily dose of 10 mg. These combined data represent a more conservative dose reduction strategy than the dosing recommendations based on CYP2D6 genotype found in the Abilify (aripiprazole) prescribing information[35] that states that known CYP2D6 PMs should be administered half of the usual dose, or 50% dose reduction, not 33% as calculated based on combined study data, thus the DPWG guideline provides additional clinical data on which to guide a practitioner's dose decisions.

PAIN MANAGEMENT
Codeine

Codeine is a prodrug opioid that must be converted into the active metabolite morphine by CYP2D6 to elicit the analgesic effect. CYP2D6 PMs do not produce adequate levels of morphine and are likely to fail therapy from lack of pain relief.[38] In a small case-controlled study, Poulsen and colleagues[39] demonstrated that, following codeine administration, neither morphine nor its metabolites could be detected in 92% of PMs, whereas at least 1 of the compounds could be detected in all EMs. Peak pain and discomfort levels were significantly reduced by codeine administration but only in normal metabolizers, thereby indicating that the analgesic effect of codeine depends on CYP2D6 activity.

Alternatively, CYP2D6 UMs produce more morphine per dose compared with EMs[40] and are at increased risk of severe, even fatal, morphine overdose.[41,42] UM patients are particularly sensitive to the respiratory depressant effects of morphine produced from codeine administration. The frequency of the UM phenotype in white patients is reported to range from 1% to 6%; however, the UM frequency in other populations vary more, ranging up to 29% (**Table 2**).[43]

FDA safety advisories have been issued in the last few years regarding the adverse event risk in patients taking codeine relative the CYP2D6 genotype. Two of these advisories detail the risk of respiratory depression in UM children and adolescents treated with codeine following tonsillectomy or adenoidectomy.[43,44] In 3 of the fatal cases involving CYP2D6 UMs, all received standard doses of codeine and all developed toxicity within 1 to 2 days of taking codeine. This rapid onset of toxicity makes the earlier identification of overdose risk even more important; even a few doses in the first day or 2 can result in fatal morphine levels. Given that drowsiness is a common side effect of codeine therapy, the recognition of expected central effects versus initial drowsiness leading to respiratory depression from overdose in the first 2 days could prove very difficult to identify clinically. Genotyping can identify these high-risk patients before the first dose is ever given.

Both the CPIC and the DPWG have published concordant guidelines based on their systematic literature reviews.[13,14] The DPWG determined a clinical evidence score of 4B for CYP2D6 PMs and 3F for CYP2D6 UMs, highlighting the documented, elevated

Table 2
Prevalence of ultrarapid metabolizers in different populations

Population	UM Genotypes/Phenotypes (↑ Activity)	Prevalence % (UM/Total number)
African or Ethiopian	UM (active duplicate genes)	29% (35/122)
African American	UM (3 active duplicate genes)	3.4% (3/87) 6.5% (60/919)
Asian	UM (active duplicate genes)	1.2% (5/400) 2%
White	UM (3 active duplicate genes)	3.6% (33/919) 6.5% (18/275)
Greek	CYP2D6*2xN/UM	6.0% (17/283)
Hungarian	UM (active duplicate genes)	1.9%
Northern European	UM (active duplicate genes)	1%–2%

Data from FDA Drug Safety Communication: Codeine use in certain children after tonsillectomy and/or adenoidectomy may lead to rare, but life-threatening adverse events or death. Available at: http://www.fda.gov/Drugs/DrugSafety/ucm313631.htm. Accessed June 1, 2016.

risk of accidental morphine overdose and death in UM patients treated with codeine.[14] The recently updated CPIC guidelines reached consensus that both CYP2D6 PMs and UMs should be considered for alternatives to codeine, such as morphine or nonopioid analgesics that do not include tramadol, and to a lesser extent, hydrocodone or oxycodone, given their reliance on the same CYP2D6 pathway for efficacy.[13,45]

CARDIOLOGY

CYP2D6 is also involved in the metabolism of several antiarrhythmic agents such as carvedilol, flecainide, metoprolol, nebivolol, propafenone, propranolol, and timolol. Variants of the CYP2D6 gene have been found to influence the response to many of these agents (ie, carvedilol, timolol, propafenone, and propranolol) but studies show the PM phenotype has a strong association with an increased risk of toxicity due to elevated plasma concentrations and prolonged half-life specifically with metoprolol.[46–48]

Metoprolol

Metoprolol is among the most commonly prescribed beta-blockers, in the top 20 prescriptions for units sold in 2013.[49] It is metabolized by CYP2D6 and studies have demonstrated a significant association of metoprolol pharmacokinetics with the CYP2D6 phenotype. A meta-analysis by Blake and colleagues[50] showed that CYP2D6 PMs have statistically higher blood concentrations, longer half-lives, and slower clearance rates than normal metabolizers (**Table 3**). Additionally, PM subjects are more likely to experience concentration-dependent side effects, including dizziness, nausea, hypotension, bradycardia, and syncope. Rau and colleagues[51] demonstrated that the higher blood concentrations attained in subjects with a CYP2D6 PM phenotype were associated with significant and persistently enhanced drug effects. In this prospective longitudinal study, 60% of PMs verses 8% of non-PMs experienced bradycardia when treated with metoprolol, leading to a 7-fold increased relative risk for bradycardia in PMs versus normal metabolizers.

After review of the published plasma concentration differences and ADR rates among different CYP2D6 phenotypes, the DPWG calculated an evidence score of

Table 3
Meta-analysis of pooled data comparing metoprolol pharmacokinetic parameters for CYP2D6 extreme phenotypes

Metoprolol pharmacokinetic	PMs vs EMs	PMs vs UMs
Plasma Concentration	2.3-fold higher	5.3-fold higher
AUC[a]	4.9-fold higher	13-fold higher
Elimination Half-life	2.3-fold longer	2.6-fold longer
Oral Clearance	5.9-fold lower	15-fold lower

Meta-analysis of 13 independent studies, n = 264.
[a] AUC, dose normalized area under the plasma concentration curve versus time.
Data from Blake CM, Kharasch ED, Schwab M, et al. A meta-analysis of CYP2D6 metabolizer phenotype and metoprolol pharmacokinetics. Clin Pharmacol Ther 2013;94(3):394–9.

4C for metoprolol for PMs (see **Table 1**). They calculated that the population size-weighted mean of the dose adjustment was 25% of the normal recommended dose. For clinical applicability, this translated to a dose reduction of 75% or selection of an alternative medication to treat heart failure. The recommended dose reduction of 75% for PMs normalizes the ADR risk due to the decreased drug clearance experienced by CYP2D6 PMs. An understanding that the mechanism of ADR risk is due to decreased clearance by CYP2D6 PMs allows the physician to take action based on that mechanism, that is, decrease the dose by 75% or possibly consider an alternative drug based on the significant risk profile.

For the opposite extreme phenotype, UMs, the DPWG scored the clinical relevance at 4D (see **Table 1**) due to the strong risk of therapeutic failure at standard dosages.[14] In CYP2D6 UMs, they recommend a dose titration to a maximum of 250% of the standard dose of metoprolol, or consideration of an alternative beta-blocker.

COST-EFFECTIVENESS

A current conundrum in propelling pharmacogenetic testing in clinical practice is resolving cost-effectiveness of testing with reimbursement policies. Many policy holders are reluctant to commit to pharmacogenetic testing unless sufficient data exist to demonstrate cost-effectiveness of the testing. However, the economics of validating pharmacogenetic testing via randomized clinical trials has been cited as a factor hampering this process.[15] Despite this, an increasing evidence base is making a case for cost-effectiveness and improved clinical outcome when pharmacogenetic testing is incorporated into the clinic.

Costs to Treat Psychiatric Disorders

Treatment-resistant depression

Treatment-resistant depression (TRD) occurs in upwards of 50% to 60% of depressed patients[52,53] and has been estimated to cost an average of $11,000 per year to treat.[54,55] Studies have shown that 30% to 46% of depressed patients do not adequately respond to their initial antidepressant and that discontinuation of the first-line antidepressant therapy is a major determinant for which patients are likely to become treatment resistant.[54] Russell and colleagues[56] (**Table 4**) demonstrated that as depressed patients are put through more medication changes and/or additions, the costs to treat these individuals more than doubles. These data also demonstrate that TRD doubles total health costs due to increased outpatient, inpatient, and pharmaceutical costs, and accrues health costs that are nearly 3-fold greater than

Table 4				
Annual costs associated with treatment-resistant depression				
	Total Health Costs		Depression-Only Health Costs	
	Non-TRD[a]	TRD[b]	Non-TRD	TRD
Russell, 2004 (n = 7737)	$6852	$13,980	$1668	$4608
Crown, 2002 (n = 3370)	$6512	$42,344	$1455	$28,001

[a] Non-TRD defined by 2 or fewer medications and/or medication changes.
[b] TRD defined by multiple recurrences, treatment failures, and 2 to 8 medications and/or regimen changes.
Data from Russell JM, Hawkins K, Ozminkowski RJ, et al. The cost consequences of treatment-resistant depression. J Clin Psychiatry 2004;65(3):341–7; and Crown WH, Finkelstein S, Berndt ER, et al. The impact of treatment-resistant depression on health care utilization and costs. J Clin Psychiatry 2002;63(11):963–71.

non-TRD depressed patients. Crown and colleagues additionally showed that compared with non-TRD depressed patients, TRD patients are twice as likely to be hospitalized, leading to a 6-fold increase in total medical costs, and a 19-fold increase in total depression-related costs (see **Table 4**).[54] Based on the available body of literature, it is increasingly clear that patients with TRD have discernibly different patterns of illness and treatment, compared with patients who respond to initial antidepressant treatment. In summary, patients with TRD are more costly and difficult to treat, which underscores the importance of early identification for safe and effective long-term treatment.

SSRIs are the most common initial antidepressant prescription.[54] Patients who display TRD are more likely to be switched to or augmented with a TCA. Many SSRIs and nearly all TCAs depend on CYP2D6. Safety of TCAs is strongly correlated with CYP2D6 genotype (see **Table 1**). The risk of adverse events in CYP2D6 PMs taking TCAs at standard doses has been extensively reviewed and recommended dose modifications based on genotype (see previous discussion). In short, increased half-life of a CYP2D6-dependent drug in the blood due to decreased elimination increases risk of toxicity, which can be placated by awareness of patient phenotype and appropriate dose adjustments. Reduction of standard doses of CYP2D6-dependent medications in CYP2D6 PM patients not only minimizes risk of ADRs but is accompanied by a substantial saving of per patient per year.

Psychoses

More than 65,000 Americans are hospitalized each year for schizophrenia and mood disorders (Centers for Disease Control and Prevention and National Institutes of Health statistics). The average length of a hospital stay for this patient subpopulation is approximately 7.1 days.[57] Studies have demonstrated that schizophrenic patients have a high probability of recurrence and hospitalization, particularly when they have had a recent relapse.[31] The probability of recurrence can range from 19% to 100%. Overall, schizophrenic patients demonstrate higher recurrent relapse risk, 4 to 5 times the annual hospitalization risk, 5 times (or higher) the annual cost, and 5 times longer hospital stays (**Table 5**). The ability to select the safest and most efficacious antipsychotic medications for these patients is critical to decrease the staggering risks associated with treatment failure, relapse, and hospitalization costs.

Many of the most commonly prescribed medications used to treat schizophrenia and related psychoses, such as risperidone, haloperidol, and aripiprazole, are metabolized by CYP2D6. Chou and colleagues[25] performed a study to determine what impact CYP2D6 genotyping would have on outcome and costs associated with severe

Table 5
Annualized hospitalization rates and costs associated with schizophrenic relapse

	No Recent Relapse			Recent Relapse		
	Hospitalization Risk[a]	Hospitalization Cost	Average Length of Stay	Hospitalization Risk	Hospitalization Cost	Average Length of Stay
Liu, 2012	12%	$7,649[b]	—	38%[c]	$73,549[b]	—
Ascher-Svanum, 2010	14%	$7786	9.84 d	51%	$38,104	51.24 d

[a] Statistics represent percentage of relapsed patients.
[b] Annual cost derived from Clinical Antipsychotic Trials of Intervention Effectiveness (CATIE) calculated by (days hospitalized × daily rate)/(day in phase/365), white paper.
[c] Survival analysis from CATIE Phase 1.

Data from Liu Q, Ramsey TL, Meltzer HY, et al. Sulfotransferase 4A1 haplotype 1 (SULT4A1-1) is associated with decreased hospitalization events in antipsychotic-treated patients with schizophrenia. Prim Care Companion CNS Disord 2012;14(3): [pii:PCC.11m01293]; and Ascher-Svanum H, Zhu B, Faries DE, et al. The cost of relapse and the predictors of relapse in the treatment of schizophrenia. BMC Psychiatry 2010;10:2.

mental illness. The study examined the influence of 2D6 variants on ADRs, hospital stays, and total costs over a 1-year period. The investigators found that patients genotyped as CYP2D6 PMs who were taking medications metabolized by CYP2D6 suffered more ADRs than both CYP2D6 normal metabolizers taking CYP2D6-dependent medications and CYP2D6 PMs taking non-CYP2D6 metabolized medications.[25] Thus, identification of patients with a CYP2D6 PM phenotype can risk-stratify patients for selection of non-CYP2D6–dependent medications (eg, quetiapine, lurasidone, or others) to reduce the increased risk burden in the PM patients.

The previously discussed study also demonstrated that PM patients taking CYP2D6-dependent medications stay an average of 7 days longer in hospital (24 days per year vs 17 days per year), at an average annual increased cost of $4000 to $6000 compared with normal metabolizers. The investigators noted that their cost calculations were likely underestimated because the average cost of a hospital bed at the study site (Eastern State, KY, USA) was roughly one-third the national average cost ($360 per day vs $1000 per day). Therefore, the investigators imply that the total cost burden may be 3 times higher than actually reported. The investigators also estimated that for CY2D6 genotyping to be cost-effective, the cost to treat PM versus normal metabolizer patients should differ by $2000 to $3000, which is well within the range of annual estimated costs (see **Table 5**).

In 2013, Herbild and colleagues[58] compared the annual cost to treat schizophrenic patients with and without pharmacogenetic testing intervention that included genotyping with CYP2D6 and CYP2C19. They modeled 2 scenarios. The first model that compared pharmacogenetic intervention to no pharmacogenetic intervention (eg, standard of care) demonstrated that total costs to treat the control group were higher than the total costs to treat the group receiving the pharmacogenetic intervention, and that most of those costs were in the psychiatric care sector (**Table 6**). The second model compared the effect of pharmacogenetic intervention on treatment costs between subjects with different genotypes (eg, extreme metabolizers vs normal metabolizers in which extreme metabolizers were those with CYP2D6 PM and UM phenotypes). In model 2, it was found that extreme metabolizers incur 177% higher total costs than normal metabolizers, and that these cost differences can be reduced by 48% using pharmacogenetic testing intervention (trend, $P = .06$). Furthermore, when the data focused on the costs incurred for psychiatric care, extreme

Table 6
Annual costs per patient to treat schizophrenia with and without pharmacogenetic intervention

Mean Costs	Control Group	Pharmacogenetic Intervention Group	Difference
Total Costs[a]	$27,350	$23,361	$4000
Psychiatric Care Costs	$21,670	$17,891	$4000
Extreme Metabolizers[b]	$67,064	$20,532	$46,000

n = 209.
[a] Costs calculated for a period of 1 year after inclusion in the study in dollars. Total costs include primary care services, secondary care services, psychiatric hospital care services, and pharmaceuticals.
[b] Mean psychiatric care costs for PMs and UMs.
Data from Herbild L, Andersen SE, Werge T, et al. Does pharmacogenetic testing for CYP450 2D6 and 2C19 among patients with diagnoses within the schizophrenic spectrum reduce treatment costs? Basic Clin Pharmacol Toxicol 2013;113(4):266–72.

metabolizers were found to incur 239% higher psychiatric costs than normal metabolizers, and that these costs could be reduced to 28% with pharmacogenetic testing intervention (significant, $P = .004$). Overall, cost within the confines of this model equated to $67,064 for extreme metabolizers, which could be reduced to $20,532 with pharmacogenetic testing. It is also important to note that the cost to genotype each subject in the group did not result in higher overall costs. In fact, modeling 2 different prices of testing ($179 to $410) did not alter the magnitude of the estimates. The statistical levels actually improved with higher costs (see **Table 6**) in which the cost table was based on the $179 test cost. In summary, costs to treat schizophrenia in extreme metabolizers are higher than the costs to treat normal metabolizers, and identification of and genotypic-specific intervention for extreme metabolizers reduces treatment costs among these patients.

A detailed economic calculation based on the impact of CYP2D6 genotype and haloperidol pharmacokinetics and treatment outcome revealed that dose adjustment based on genotype could help avoid EPS, amounting to cost savings in the end via the avoidance of severe ADRs. This study demonstrated that 80% of CYPD6 PMs experience significant EPS but that genotype-based dose adjustments could lower this percentage to 16%, the percentage of EMs and IMs that experience EPS following haloperidol.[33] The investigators calculated that genotyping 2% patients undergoing haloperidol treatment would be sufficient to avoid 1 severe ADR. In summary, the logic follows that if the CYP2D6 PM phenotype occurs in 7% of the population, then 70 out of 1000 treated patients would be PMs, and 56 patients (80%) would be at risk of significant EPS. If this percentage were reduced to 16% (normalizing risk compared with that seen in normal CYP2D6 metabolizers), then 45 of those patients could potentially benefit from dose adjustments to help avoid EPS. Based on parameters of the economics of genotyping to the total number of patients to treat, the number of patients needed to genotype to avoid 1 severe ADR in this scenario would be $1/(45/1000) = 22$ patients. At the 2016 Centers for Medicare and Medicaid Services fee schedule of $450 for CYP2D6 ($450 \times 22$) it would cost $9900 to avoid 1 severe ADR. Considering the average cost to treat a nontherapeutic relapsed patient (treatment failure or worsening symptoms, or discontinuation due to ADR) is $38,104 or more (see **Table 5**), the estimated cost of genotyping, $9900, to avoid 1 severe ADR would more than adequately justify the coverage of genotyping expense.

Cost to Treat Heart Failure: Metoprolol

In 2008, the estimated total cost of heart failure (HF) in the United States was $34.8 billion, with the greatest share being due to hospitalizations. The average cost associated with an heart failure hospitalization is $10,000. While approximately 14% of Medicare beneficiaries have heart failure, they account for 43% of Medicare spending.

The risk of heart failure increases by 2 and 3 fold respectively in hypertensive men and women. The Metoprolol CR/XL Randomised Intervention Trial in Congestive Heart Failure (MERIT-HF) trial (1999) demonstrated that treatment with metoprolol significantly affected clinical outcomes by decreasing (1) mortality rate by 34%, (2) sudden death by 41%, (3) death due to heart failure by 49%, and (4) hospitalizations by 36%.[59] More specifically, 134 fewer subjects treated with metoprolol versus placebo were hospitalized for worsening heart failure. Using the average estimate of $10,000 per hospitalization, the use of metoprolol equates to a savings of at least $1.3 million. Withdrawal of beta-blocker therapy due to adverse events is also associated with increased mortality. In the same study, worsening heart failure, bradycardia, dizziness, and hypotension were among the common reasons for metoprolol withdrawal.

Taken together, the combined data demonstrate a continuum of risk in which PMs have a 7-fold higher risk of ADRs. ADRs increase risk of metoprolol discontinuation and heart failure patients not therapeutically managed with metoprolol are at increased risk of hospitalizations and death. Therefore, identifying patients at increased risk of therapeutic failure, either due to lack of efficacy (UMs) or due to discontinuation from adverse events (PMs), can significantly affect mortality rate or overall cost to the health care system, and genotyping can identify patients at the beginning of this continuum of risk.

DISCUSSION AND SUMMARY

The CYP2D6 enzyme, responsible for the metabolism of a significant proportion of all prescribed medications, is recognized as among the most important biomarkers of drug response. Guidelines for optimizing treatment via pharmacogenetic testing of CYP2D6 are available for several antidepressive agents, antipsychotics, and pain medications. It is understood that, although CYP2D6 is involved in the metabolism of many prescription medications, there is more to drug response than just metabolism. Some medications are metabolized by more than 1 enzyme with genetic variability. Many medications are also affected by differences in pharmacodynamic response genes, such as those that encode drug receptors, drug transporters, and cellular membrane pumps. The inherited combinations of pharmacokinetic and pharmacodynamic drug response modulators are essential to ultimately predict how a patient is likely to respond to a particular medication. For this reason, pharmacogenetic panels are important for eliciting the most useful medication sensitivity information and to provide insight into alternative treatment options. For example, a patient identified as a PM for 1 metabolic pathway, may be a candidate for a medication metabolized by another pathway for which that patient has been identified as a normal (extensive) metabolizer. One of the difficulties with pharmacogenetic testing panels is the complexity of the results. Recent studies in which combinatorial guidance was provided along with pharmacogenetic panel results revealed that when clinicians made genotype-guided selections, subjects improved adherence and saved $1035.60 in total drug spending over a 1-year period compared with unguided matched controls.[60,61] More striking was when clinicians made medication selections based on gene-guided reports, subjects saved an average of $2774.53 per year compared with the subjects who are not genotype-guided, with anxiety disorder representing the largest savings of $6874.69 per year.[61] Interestingly, 1 in 5 subjects in the genotype-guided group was taking 1 less medication by the end of the study period compared with the group that was not genotype-guided.

Thus, personalized medicine in the form of pharmacogenetic testing and genotype-guided support has been demonstrated to improve drug efficacy, decrease side effect risk, decrease medical costs, and reduce polypharmacy. CYP2D6 is a significant contributor to that outcome, whereas polypharmacy risk is yet another factor. The combinatorial assessment of multigene and polypharmacy interaction risks provides a more complete picture of a patient's true medication risk burden. A panel-based approach accounting for drug-gene and drug-drug interactions improves sensitivity to detect high-risk drugs, identify safer doses, more efficacious alternatives, and ultimately improve health care costs.

REFERENCES

1. U.S. Food and Drug Administration: table of pharmacogenomic biomarkers in drug labeling. 2015. Available at: http://www.fda.gov/Drugs/ScienceResearch/ResearchAreas/Pharmacogenetics/ucm083378.htm. Accessed June 1, 2016.

2. Clinical Pharmacogenetics Implementation Consortium. Available at: www. cpicpgx.org. Accessed June 1, 2016.

3. The pharmacogenomics knowledgebase: dosing guidelines - CPIC. 2015-16. Available at: www.pharmgkb.org. Accessed June 1, 2016.

4. Evans WE, Relling MV. Pharmacogenomics: translating functional genomics into rational therapeutics. Science 1999;286(5439):487–91.

5. Eichelbaum M, Ingelman-Sundberg M, Evans WE. Pharmacogenomics and individualized drug therapy. Annu Rev Med 2006;57:119–37.

6. Zanger UM, Raimundo S, Eichelbaum M. Cytochrome P450 2D6: overview and update on pharmacology, genetics, biochemistry. Naunyn Schmiedebergs Arch Pharmacol 2004;369(1):23–37.

7. Samer CF, Lorenzini KI, Rollason V, et al. Applications of CYP450 testing in the clinical setting. Mol Diagn Ther 2013;17(3):165–84.

8. Hicks JK, Swen JJ, Thorn CF, et al. Clinical Pharmacogenetics Implementation Consortium guideline for CYP2D6 and CYP2C19 genotypes and dosing of tricyclic antidepressants. Clin Pharmacol Ther 2013;93(5):402–8.

9. Bradford LD. CYP2D6 allele frequency in European Caucasians, Asians, Africans and their descendants. Pharmacogenomics 2002;3(2):229–43.

10. Hicks JK, Swen JJ, Gaedigk A. Challenges in CYP2D6 phenotype assignment from genotype data: a critical assessment and call for standardization. Curr Drug Metab 2014;15(2):218–32.

11. CPIC: Final terms for the CPIC Term Standardization Project 2016(4/27/2016). 2016. Available at: https://cpicpgx.org/wpcontent/uploads/2016/01/CPIC_term_standardization_project_final_terms.pdf. Accessed June 1, 2016.

12. Ingelman-Sundberg M, Oscarson M, Mclellan RA. Polymorphic human cytochrome P450 enzymes: an opportunity for individualized drug treatment. Trends Pharmacol Sci 1999;20(8):342–9.

13. Crews KR, Gaedigk A, Dunnenberger HM, et al. Clinical Pharmacogenetics Implementation Consortium (CPIC) guidelines for codeine therapy in the context of cytochrome P450 2D6 (CYP2D6) genotype. Clin Pharmacol Ther 2012;91(2): 321–6.

14. Swen JJ, Nijenhuis M, De Boer A, et al. Pharmacogenetics: from bench to byte–an update of guidelines. Clin Pharmacol Ther 2011;89(5):662–73.

15. Walk EE. Improving the power of diagnostics in the era of targeted therapy and personalized healthcare. Curr Opin Drug Discov Devel 2010;13(2):226–34.

16. Ventola CL. Pharmacogenomics in clinical practice: reality and expectations. P T 2011;36(7):412–50.

17. Hicks JK, Bishop JR, Sangkuhl K, et al. Clinical Pharmacogenetics Implementation Consortium (CPIC) guideline for CYP2D6 and CYP2C19 genotypes and dosing of selective serotonin reuptake inhibitors. Clin Pharmacol Ther 2015; 98(2):127–34.

18. Shams ME, Arneth B, Hiemke C, et al. CYP2D6 polymorphism and clinical effect of the antidepressant venlafaxine. J Clin Pharm Ther 2006;31(5):493–502.

19. Grasmader K, Verwohlt PL, Rietschel M, et al. Impact of polymorphisms of cytochrome-P450 isoenzymes 2C9, 2C19 and 2D6 on plasma concentrations and clinical effects of antidepressants in a naturalistic clinical setting. Eur J Clin Pharmacol 2004;60(5):329–36.

20. Mcalpine DE, O'kane DJ, Black JL, et al. Cytochrome P450 2D6 genotype variation and venlafaxine dosage. Mayo Clin Proc 2007;82(9):1065–8.

21. Lessard E, Yessine MA, Hamelin BA, et al. Influence of CYP2D6 activity on the disposition and cardiovascular toxicity of the antidepressant agent venlafaxine in humans. Pharmacogenetics 1999;9(4):435–43.

22. Koski A, Ojanpera I, Sistonen J, et al. A fatal doxepin poisoning associated with a defective CYP2D6 genotype. Am J Forensic Med Pathol 2007;28(3):259–61.

23. Baldessarini RJ, Tarazi FI. Pharmacotherapy of psychosis and mania. In: Brunton L, Lazo J, Parker K, editors. Goodman & Gilman's the pharmacological basis of therapeutics. 11th edition. New York: McGraw-Hill; 2005. p. 461–500.

24. Risperdal (R) [package insert]. Janssen Pharmaceuticals, Titusville, NJ. 2014.

25. Chou WH, Yan FX, De Leon J, et al. Extension of a pilot study: impact from the cytochrome P450 2D6 polymorphism on outcome and costs associated with severe mental illness. J Clin Psychopharmacol 2000;20(2):246–51.

26. De Leon J, Susce MT, Pan RM, et al. The CYP2D6 poor metabolizer phenotype may be associated with risperidone adverse drug reactions and discontinuation. J Clin Psychiatry 2005;66(1):15–27.

27. De Leon J, Susce MT, Pan RM, et al. Polymorphic variations in GSTM1, GSTT1, PgP, CYP2D6, CYP3A5, and dopamine D2 and D3 receptors and their association with tardive dyskinesia in severe mental illness. J Clin Psychopharmacol 2005;25(5):448–56.

28. Kohnke MD, Griese EU, Stosser D, et al. Cytochrome P450 2D6 deficiency and its clinical relevance in a patient treated with risperidone. Pharmacopsychiatry 2002; 35(3):116–8.

29. Llerena A, Berecz R, Dorado P, et al. QTc interval, CYP2D6 and CYP2C9 genotypes and risperidone plasma concentrations. J Psychopharmacol 2004;18(2): 189–93.

30. Scordo MG, Spina E, Facciola G, et al. Cytochrome P450 2D6 genotype and steady state plasma levels of risperidone and 9-hydroxyrisperidone. Psychopharmacology (Berl) 1999;147(3):300–5.

31. Vasudeva S, Narendra Kumar MS, Sekhar KC. Duration of first admission and its relation to the readmission rate in a psychiatry hospital. Indian J Psychiatry 2009; 51(4):280–4.

32. Ascher-Svanum H, Zhu B, Faries DE, et al. The cost of relapse and the predictors of relapse in the treatment of schizophrenia. BMC Psychiatry 2010;10:2.

33. Brockmoller J, Kirchheiner J, Schmider J, et al. The impact of the CYP2D6 polymorphism on haloperidol pharmacokinetics and on the outcome of haloperidol treatment. Clin Pharmacol Ther 2002;72(4):438–52.

34. U.S. Pharmaceutical Sales 2013. Available at: http://www.drugs.com/stats/top100/2013/sales. Accessed June 1, 2016.

35. Abilify (R) [package insert]. Tokyo: Otsuka Pharmaceutical Co., Ltd; 2016.

36. Surja AAS, Reynolds KK, Linder MW, et al. Pharmacogenetic testing of CYP2D6 in patients with aripiprazole-related extrapyramidal symptoms: a case-control study. Pers Med 2008;5(4):361–5.

37. Swen JJ, Van Der Straaten T, Wessels JA, et al. Feasibility of pharmacy-initiated pharmacogenetic screening for CYP2D6 and CYP2C19. Eur J Clin Pharmacol 2012;68(4):363–70.

38. Reynolds KK, Ramey-Hartung B, Jortani SA. The value of CYP2D6 and OPRM1 pharmacogenetic testing for opioid therapy. Clin Lab Med 2008;28(4):581–98.

39. Poulsen L, Brosen K, Arendt-Nielsen L, et al. Codeine and morphine in extensive and poor metabolizers of sparteine: pharmacokinetics, analgesic effect and side effects. Eur J Clin Pharmacol 1996;51(3–4):289–95.

40. Kirchheiner J, Schmidt H, Tzvetkov M, et al. Pharmacokinetics of codeine and its metabolite morphine in ultra-rapid metabolizers due to CYP2D6 duplication. Pharmacogenomics J 2007;7(4):257–65.
41. Gasche Y, Daali Y, Fathi M, et al. Codeine intoxication associated with ultrarapid CYP2D6 metabolism. N Engl J Med 2004;351(27):2827–31.
42. Ciszkowski C, Madadi P, Phillips MS, et al. Codeine, ultrarapid-metabolism genotype, and postoperative death. N Engl J Med 2009;361(8):827–8.
43. U.S. Food and Drug Administration: FDA Drug Safety Communication: Codeine use in certain children after tonsillectomy and/or adenoidectomy may lead to rare, but life-threatening adverse events or death. 2012. Available at: http://www.fda.gov/Drugs/DrugSafety/ucm313631.htm. Accessed June 1, 2016.
44. U.S. Food and Drug Administration: FDA Drug Safety Communication: Safety review update of codeine use in children; new boxed warning and contraindication on use after tonsillectomy and/or adenoidectomy. 2013. Available at: http://www.fda.gov/Drugs/DrugSafety/ucm339112.htm. Accessed June 1, 2016.
45. Crews KR, Gaedigk A, Dunnenberger HM, et al. Clinical Pharmacogenetics Implementation Consortium guidelines for cytochrome P450 2D6 genotype and codeine therapy: 2014 update. Clin Pharmacol Ther 2014;95(4):376–82.
46. Cascorbi I. Pharmacogenetics of cytochrome p4502D6: genetic background and clinical implication. Eur J Clin Invest 2003;33(Suppl 2):17–22.
47. Rogers JF, Nafziger AN, Bertino JS Jr. Pharmacogenetics affects dosing, efficacy, and toxicity of cytochrome P450-metabolized drugs. Am J Med 2002;113(9):746–50.
48. Wuttke H, Rau T, Heide R, et al. Increased frequency of cytochrome P450 2D6 poor metabolizers among patients with metoprolol-associated adverse effects. Clin Pharmacol Ther 2002;72(4):429–37.
49. Top 100 drugs for 2013 by units sold. Available at http://www.drugs.com/stats/top100/2013/units. Accessed June 1, 2016.
50. Blake CM, Kharasch ED, Schwab M, et al. A meta-analysis of CYP2D6 metabolizer phenotype and metoprolol pharmacokinetics. Clin Pharmacol Ther 2013;94(3):394–9.
51. Rau T, Wuttke H, Michels LM, et al. Impact of the CYP2D6 genotype on the clinical effects of metoprolol: a prospective longitudinal study. Clin Pharmacol Ther 2009;85(3):269–72.
52. Fava M. Diagnosis and definition of treatment-resistant depression. Biol Psychiatry 2003;53(8):649–59.
53. Fava M, Davidson KG. Definition and epidemiology of treatment-resistant depression. Psychiatr Clin North Am 1996;19(2):179–200.
54. Crown WH, Finkelstein S, Berndt ER, et al. The impact of treatment-resistant depression on health care utilization and costs. J Clin Psychiatry 2002;63(11):963–71.
55. Corey-Lisle PK, Birnbaum HG, Greenberg PE, et al. Identification of a claims data "signature" and economic consequences for treatment-resistant depression. J Clin Psychiatry 2002;63(8):717–26.
56. Russell JM, Hawkins K, Ozminkowski RJ, et al. The cost consequences of treatment-resistant depression. J Clin Psychiatry 2004;65(3):341–7.
57. Liu Q, Ramsey TL, Meltzer HY, et al. Sulfotransferase 4A1 haplotype 1 (SULT4A1–1) is associated with decreased hospitalization events in antipsychotic-treated patients with schizophrenia. Prim Care Companion CNS Disord 2012;14(3) [pii: PCC.11m01293].

58. Herbild L, Andersen SE, Werge T, et al. Does pharmacogenetic testing for CYP450 2D6 and 2C19 among patients with diagnoses within the schizophrenic spectrum reduce treatment costs? Basic Clin Pharmacol Toxicol 2013;113(4): 266–72.
59. Effect of metoprolol CR/XL in chronic heart failure: Metoprolol CR/XL Randomised Intervention Trial in Congestive Heart Failure (MERIT-HF). Lancet 1999;353(9169): 2001–7.
60. Winner JG, Carhart JM, Altar CA, et al. A prospective, randomized, double-blind study assessing the clinical impact of integrated pharmacogenomic testing for major depressive disorder. Discov Med 2013;16(89):219–27.
61. Winner JG, Carhart JM, Altar CA, et al. Combinatorial pharmacogenomic guidance for psychiatric medications reduces overall pharmacy costs in a 1 year prospective evaluation. Curr Med Res Opin 2015;31(9):1633–43.

The Pharmacist's Perspective on Pharmacogenetics Implementation

Frederick Weitendorf, RN, RPh[a,b], Kristen K. Reynolds, PhD[b,c],*

KEYWORDS

- Pharmacogenetics • Pharmacokinetics • Pharmacodynamics
- Drug–gene interaction • Personalized medicine

KEY POINTS

- Pharmacists have the chance to apply and incorporate drug knowledge in collaboration with physicians and other health care providers using pharmacogenetics.
- This will not be just in a general broad context, but will be personalized for each patient reflecting that patient's drug–gene metabolic pathway.
- Patients with this approach benefit with enhanced therapeutic outcomes that could lead to more streamlined drug approaches, fewer follow-up visits, cost savings, and shorter times to achieve therapeutic outcomes.
- Drug–gene metabolic pathways will allow the providers to avoid drug failures, customize doses and schedules, alert drugs using the same pathway, and prevent duplication of therapies.
- The time will arrive when no medication order can be processed without the knowledge of the patient's drug–gene metabolic pathway.

INTRODUCTION

Every pharmacist has a goal to maximize medication therapy success and minimize medication therapy failure. Currently, pharmacists review the patient's renal status, allergies, hepatic function, weight, gender, and other parameters to optimize medication response and minimize and adverse drug reactions that may occur. This all occurs within an institutional drug formulary with the goal of successful patient outcomes and

[a] Robley Rex Veterans Affairs Medical Center, 800 Zorn Avenue, Louisville, KY 40206, USA;
[b] PGXL Laboratories, 201 East Jefferson Street, Suite 309, Louisville, KY 40202, USA;
[c] Department of Pathology and Laboratory Medicine, University of Louisville School of Medicine, 627 South Preston Street, Louisville, KY 40292, USA
* Corresponding author. PGXL Laboratories, 201 East Jefferson Street, Suite 309, Louisville, KY 40202.
E-mail address: kreynolds@pgxlab.com

Clin Lab Med 36 (2016) 543–556
http://dx.doi.org/10.1016/j.cll.2016.05.009
0272-2712/16/$ – see front matter © 2016 Elsevier Inc. All rights reserved.

labmed.theclinics.com

cost controls. Pharmacogenetics adds another tool for the pharmacist to enhance successful outcomes and minimize untoward effects. Knowing a patient's drug–gene metabolic pathway allows the pharmacist to aid the provider with that ability to avoid medications metabolized by the liver that will not result in the desired outcome. Adverse drug reactions (ADRs) are one of the leading causes of death in the United States.[1] If the drug–gene metabolic pathways are identified before implementation, up to almost 60% of ADR risk could be identified and managed[2] (**Table 1**). Having this knowledge gives the provider and the pharmacist the ability to select medications that would give a greater chance of success and avoid those medications that genetically would be impaired. This ability to identify patient variability genetically helps to illuminate why certain patients respond better than others and also why others fail to achieve the desired effects. This variability then can be viewed as a function of the patient's unique genetic makeup and used to enhance the personalization of medications. The impact is better medication selection, resulting in safer administration, quicker drug response, and cost savings by avoiding other risky medications and fewer follow-up provider visits to monitor outcomes. Idiosyncratic reactions now can be explained partially with an increasing knowledge of the drug–gene metabolic pathways, reflecting the variations that exist among individuals. This personalized approach to medicine reflecting pharmacogenetics gives the pharmacist a special opportunity to understand on a molecular level each patient and their predicted response.

PHARMACOGENETICS IS MORE THAN JUST DRUG METABOLISM

Pharmacogenetic variants affect modulators of both pharmacokinetic (PK) and pharmacodynamic (PD) processes, and have very different consequences on drug safety and efficacy. Pharmacology is broken down into 2 equal sides for every drug: the PK effect and the PD response. Genetic variants in both PK and PD mechanisms can affect drug safety and efficacy, but they do so by very different mechanisms.

Pharmacokinetics

PK is what the body does to the drug. It is the process of drug disposition—absorption, distribution, metabolism, and excretion—that sets the concentration of drug delivered to the target receptor site. Absorption reflects the administration of the drug by injectable, oral, subcutaneous, rectal, and transdermal routes with the fraction of drug available in systemic circulation termed *bioavailability*. If the drug undergoes metabolism or elimination before entering the circulation, or absorption is reduced, then the bioavailability is reduced. When drugs are given by rapid intravenous injection, the peak concentration occurs earlier and higher than when the same dose is administered by a nonintravenous route. Chemical properties such as insolubility, destruction at the site of administration, or incomplete release from the drug medication form may also reduce the amount absorbed. Deliberately slowing absorption is the goal of extended release or sustained release formulations, which results in minimizing plasma drug level fluctuations between doses. A *steady state* occurs with continuous intravenous infusion whereas, in oral administration, plasma concentrations vary during the dosing interval and steady state is achieved in 5 half-lives when given consistently. The distribution of drugs for a 70-kg human is about 20 L extracellular water, blood volume of about 5.5 L, and a plasma volume of 3 L. Many drug factors can affect volumes of distribution. For example, tricyclic antidepressants and digoxin are highly bound to tissues for a high volume of distribution, whereas warfarin is protein bound in plasma and reflects a much lower volume.

Table 1
Top 10 medications leading to ADRs requiring hospitalization

Rank	Drug or Drug Class	Individual Drugs	Adverse Reactions
1	*NSAIDS*	Aspirin, diclofenac, ibuprofen, rofecoxib, celecoxib, ketoprofen, naproxen	GI bleeding, peptic ulceration, hemorrhagic stroke, renal impairment, wheezing, rash
2	Diuretics	Furosemide, bendroflumethiazide, bumetanide, spironolactone, amiloride, metolazone, indaptamide	Renal impairment, hypotension, electrolyte disturbances, gout
3	*Warfarin*	—	GI bleeding, hematuria, high INR, hematoma
4	ACE inhibitors/ all receptor antagonists	Ramipril, enalapril, captopril, lisinopril, irbesartan, losartan, perindopril	Renal impairment, hypotension, electrolyte disturbances, angioedema
5	*Antidepressants*	Fluoxetine, paroxetine, amitriptyline, citalopram, lithium, venlafaxine, dosulepin	Confusion, hypotension, constipation, GI bleed, hyponatremia
6	*Beta-blockers*	Atenolol, propranolol, sotalol, bisoprolol, metoprolol, carvedilol	Bradycardia, heart block, hypotension, wheezing
7	*Opiates*	Morphine, dihydrocodeine, co-codamol, tramadol, co-dydramol, fentanyl	Constipation, vomiting, confusion, urinary retention
8	Digoxin	—	Symptomatic toxicity
9	Prednisolone	—	Gastritis, GI bleeding, hyperglycemia, osteoporotic fracture
10	*Clopidogrel*	—	GI bleeding

Drugs or drug classes in italic are known to be affected by pharmacogenetic variants for which clinical diagnostics tests are available to identify patients with genetic ADR risk factors.

Abbreviations: ACE, angiotensin-converting enzyme; ADR, adverse drug reaction; GI, gastrointestinal; INT, international normalized ratio; NSAID, nonsteroidal antiinflammatory drug.

Adapted from Pirmohamed M, James S, Meakin S, et al. Adverse drug reactions as cause of admission to hospital: prospective analysis of 18 820 patients. BMJ 2004;329:17.

Drug loading doses attempt to achieve faster drug elevations, but the true steady state is reflected in the elimination half-life. Over time, drug elimination reduces the amount of drug burden. How fast or slowly a drug is cleared determines the dose rate required to achieve stable therapeutic blood concentrations of the drug. The reduction in drug levels results owing to clearance is driven by both metabolism and excretion. Diseases, drug interactions, and genetic variations—for example, cytochrome P450 2D6 (CYP2D6) poor metabolizer variants—can reduce the activity of drug metabolism and lead to lower drug clearance, requiring a reduction in the drug dose to avoid undesired toxic effects (**Fig. 1**). If there is an increase in drug elimination caused by drug interaction induction, or genetic variation, so-called ultrarapid metabolizers, then an increase in the drug dose may be needed to achieve therapeutic goals. Metabolites may or may not produce similar effects as the initial (parent) drug. The metabolite may be more active or totally inactive. Prodrugs are the inactive parent drugs that must be metabolized into active metabolites, resulting in therapeutic effect. Clopidogrel (antiplatelet), tamoxifen (antiestrogen), and codeine (analgesic) are examples of prodrugs.[3] With codeine, the active metabolite morphine is produced by CYP2D6, and it is the active morphine metabolite that results in the desired analgesic effect[4–6] (**Fig. 2**). Decreased or low metabolism results in low pain relief, and rapid or enhanced metabolism may result in the conversion of toxic amounts of morphine causing respiratory depression, loss of consciousness, and in rare cases, death.[4,5,7] This illustrates the high risks that may occur with drugs depend on a single metabolic pathway. Decreased CYP2D6 activity for codeine lower the therapeutic analgesic effect and decreased activity of CYP2C19 lessens the antiplatelet effect for clopidogrel. Drug elimination that may rely on a single pathway affected by genetic variation or inhibition will lead to increased drug levels and for drugs with narrow therapeutic ranges may lead to toxicity. Those individuals with decreased function in CYP2C9 responsible for the metabolism of warfarin, will be at risk for bleeding. With gene–drug variations and drug–drug interactions elimination pathway loss or impairment could have a serious impact on drug concentrations and effects.

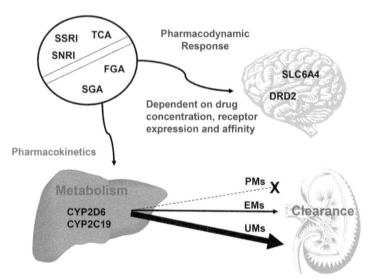

Fig. 1. Therapeutic efficacy of psychiatric medications depends on the interaction between PK and PD drug profiles. The therapeutic (PD) response to a given drug is dictated by drug occupancy of the target protein. This interaction is mediated by target number and affinity, as well as a consistent drug concentration at the target. Drug concentration is maintained by the balance of drug accumulation rate (owing to dosage) and clearance rate (owing to metabolism). Pharmacogenetic variants in a PD pathway will affect the concentration dependency of the target by altering protein affinity or expression, whereas variants in a metabolic PK pathway will alter clearance rate, drug half-life, and concentration at the target. CYP2D6, cytochrome P450 2D6; CYP2C19, cytochrome P450 2C19; DRD2, dopamine D2 receptor; EM, extensive metabolizer; FGA, first-generation antipsychotic; PM, poor metabolizer; SGA, second-generation antipsychotic; SLC6A4, serotonin transporter; SSRI, selective serotonin reuptake inhibitor; SNRI, serotonin-norepinephrine reuptake inhibitor; TCA, tricyclic antidepressant; UMs, ultrarapid metabolizers. (*Adapted from* Ramey-Hartung B, El-Mallakh RS, Reynolds KK. Pharmacogenetic testing in schizophrenia and posttraumatic stress disorder. Clin Lab Med 2008;28:634; with permission.)

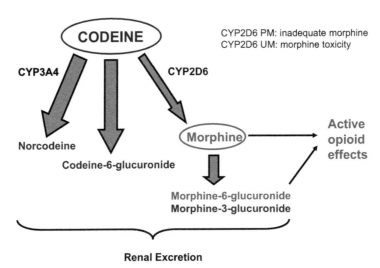

Fig. 2. Codeine metabolism. Roughly 90% of a codeine dose is metabolized to inactive compounds by cytochrome P3A4. The other 10% of a codeine dose is metabolized to the active component morphine via cytochrome P450 2D6. All are eventually excreted by the kidneys. Blue = inactive compounds; red = active metabolites. PM, poor metabolizer; UM, ultrarapid metabolizer. (*Adapted from* Reynolds KK, Ramey-Hartung B, Jortani SA. The Value of CYP2D6 and OPRM1 pharmacogenetic testing for opioid therapy. Clin Lab Med 2008;28:591; with permission.)

Pharmacodynamic Partners

The PK action of titration is based on tolerance and the PD of response (see **Fig. 1**). PD is what the drug does to the body: what the therapeutic effect is, for example, analgesia for morphine, lower blood pressure for β-blockers, and so on. Every drug elicits its therapeutic PD effect by binding to its target receptor in a concentration-dependent manner. Too much drug binding the receptor can lead to toxic side effects and too little drug binding the receptor can result in a subtherapeutic response. How much concentration of drug that gets to the location of the receptor is PK dependent. However, once the drug gets there in the right concentration, the receptor has to be present and has to be able to bind the drug to elicit the desired response.

The PD response depends on the drug concentration at the target receptor site, the amount of the target produced, and how well the receptor binds the drug. Variants in genes that code for PD target proteins can affect concentration dependency and affinity, either by decreasing receptor expression or decreasing the binding capacity for the particular drug. The serotonin transporter encoded by the SLC6A4 gene is the PD target for selective serotonin receptor inhibitor (SSRI) antidepressants, whereas the dopamine receptor DRD2 is a PD target for many common antipsychotics. Variants in both genes have been associated with decreased therapeutic response to SSRIs and antipsychotic agents, respectively[8–10] (see **Fig. 1**). The presence of the SLC6A4 "short" variant confers a reduced expression of the transporter, thereby making less target for the SSRIs to bind and elicit the PD response, that is, serotonin reuptake inhibition.[8,9] Patients with SLC6A4 poor responder phenotypes demonstrate significantly lower clinical response and remission rates compared with patients with the normal responder phenotype.[8,9] Incorporation of a pharmacogenetic panel for selection of antidepressant therapy could, therefore, start with

SLC6A4 to identify good candidates for SSRIs and those who should avoid the entire class of SSRIs, whereas the PK partner CYP genotypes could be used to refine and titrate dosages.[11] For example, a patient with the SLC6A4 normal responder phenotype would be expected to have normal therapeutic response to the SSRI paroxetine, however, because of the patient's CYP2D6 poor metabolizer phenotype, he would need to be considered for a lower than average dose, possibly a 50% dose reduction, based on the recent Clinical Pharmacogenetics Implementation Consortium guideline.[11] Conversely, a patient with a CYP2D6 ultrarapid metabolizer phenotype would be expected to have higher than normal clearance of paroxetine; however, the PD response is impaired or subtherapeutic when the patient is also a SLC6A4 a poor responder or intermediate responder. Increasing the dose for the SSRI based solely on the CYP2D6 ultrarapid metabolizer status may prove ineffective and, instead, suggests selection of a non-SSRI for treatment of the patient's depression.[8,9,11] In 1 patient, the use of those PK–PD partner genes predicts a dose adjustment to an SSRI, whereas in another patients, the same gene with different phenotype predicts a class switch.

PHARMACY-GUIDED IMPLEMENTATION OF PHARMACOGENETICS INTO CLINICAL SETTINGS

Pharmacists routinely incorporate multifactorial risk assessments into patient medication plan decisions, from issues of comorbidity and polypharmacy to diet and compliance. The use of pharmacogenetic panels adds complex multigene and multidrug assessment into the approach. The pharmacist's expertise in general medication therapy management (MTM) is the natural home for incorporation of additional pharmacologic data that is dictated by the patient's unique genetic baseline drug handling characteristics. Pharmacists can implement pharmacogenetics into their practice paradigms in several clinical settings, including hospital system pharmacy and outpatient MTM clinics.

Hospital Pharmacy and the Health System Pharmacy

The pharmacist working in clinical systems related to hospitals deals with the full array of pharmaceuticals. From routine vitamin orders to complex cancer chemotherapy regimens, the pharmacist must constantly change perspectives in pharmaceutical care. This is especially true with many patients currently having polypharmacy. The goal the entire time is to maximize therapeutic outcomes and minimize therapeutic failures and adverse drug events. The practice of health system pharmacy has evolved from a dispensing function to now having the pharmacist as a collaborator with providers to provide optimal outcomes with medications. The pharmacist reviews the medication order for appropriate application, route, dose, and potential drug–drug interactions in the context of the patient's current laboratory values, outpatient medications, gender, age, weight, and any other parameters that may affect the patient. Pharmacogenetics and knowledge of drug–gene pathways adds 1 more tool to help the pharmacist achieve this goal. The pharmacist also must take into account adverse events and be able to ensure the safe, efficient, and timely administration of drugs.

ADRs are a huge burden to morbidity and mortality in the United States, with genetic differences contributing a significant portion of that risk. **Table 1** reflects the hospitalizations owing to ADRs with the drug groups in italic showing those which have known genetic component that increase ADR risk. The Food and Drug Administration's Table of Pharmacogenomic Biomarkers in Drug Labeling cites more than 130 individual drugs with some sort of genetic information contained in the drug labeling.[12]

As more drug–gene metabolic pathways are identified the result is the ability to personalize the medications for each patient. Genotyping a patient for a single indication, drug, or gene is unlikely to reveal the patient's true risk burden based on the comorbidities and polypharmacy. When the pharmacist has the knowledge based on a panel approach for drug–gene and drug–drug interactions there is an increased sensitivity to detect high-risk drugs and identify safer doses and/or more efficacious alternatives. The pharmacogenetic panels currently available in clinical laboratories vary, but include a range from PK genes like CYP2D6, CYP2C19, and CYP2C9 to PD target genes such as OPRM1 (mu-opioid receptor) and SLC6A4 (serotonin transporter).

This gives a pharmacist and incredible insight if the patient's gene-based medication risk factors are known before drug administration. In addition to the pharmacist having access to the allergies and known adverse reactions listed, pharmacogenetics alerts the pharmacist to any potential impairment of pathways and also multiple medications that use the same medication pathway that may increase the risk for adverse events. The obvious outcome of this is the ability to tailor therapy, avoiding drug failure and potential harm to the patient.

The pharmacist with knowledge of the patient's pharmacogenetic results reconciled against their medication list is able to tailor dose or selection alternative medication options to enhance therapeutic outcome. For example, a provider has initiated a written order for metoprolol of 50 mg orally twice daily for a β-blocker–naïve patient. The gene–drug profile reveals that the patient is a CYP2D6 intermediate metabolizer, which is consistent with reduced CYP2D6 metabolic activity. This patient has a greater risk of a toxic side effect from decreased clearance, and thus, may respond to lower doses. The Dutch Pharmacogenetics Working Group guideline for metoprolol dose modification in CYP2D6 intermediate metabolizers is a 50% dose reduction from standard dosing.[3] In collaboration with the provider, the pharmacist may suggest, in the context of other medications, a 50% dose reduction to metoprolol 25 mg orally twice daily, potentially avoiding bradycardia or a decrease in blood pressure. The pharmacist also has the insight to identify other medications that may likewise rely on CYP2D6, which would further exacerbate side effect risk with metoprolol via competitive clearance.

Pain management in the hospitalized patient is another area primed for pharmacogenetic intervention. Many patients require the use of opiates, nonsteroidal antiinflammatory drugs, or other pain medications during their stay and beyond discharge. Certain widely used opiate formulations contain prodrugs, hydrocodone and oxycodone, that depend of CYP2D6 metabolic pathway for conversion to hydromorphone and oxymorphone, respectively. Using an example patient with known CYP2D6 poor metabolizer status, the inability to convert the prodrug oxycodone to the active metabolite significantly reduces the patient's ability to achieve pain relief. Active forms of opiates would increase the chance for pain relief, but with opiates now OPRM1, the gene coding for the mu opioid receptor, must be taken into account for the opiate to bind to the receptor to elicit pain relief. In those patients that are OPRM1 poor responders, the decrease in receptor availability may significantly increase opiate dose requirements.[6,13] For example, the nurse calls the pharmacist to inquire why, after dose increases of hydrocodone 5 mg/acetaminophen 300 mg to hydrocodone 7.5 mg/acetaminophen 300 mg, the patient continues to communicate little or no relief. The pharmacist finds the patient is a poor metabolizer and an OPRM1 poor opioid responder. The most likely explanation is inadequate conversion of hydrocodone to hydromorphone coupled with the insight of also being an OPRM1 poor responder that may require higher than normal opiate dosing. In collaboration with the provider, the pharmacist could recommend hydromorphone as an alternative with the caveat that a higher than normal titration upward may need to be done for this patient to receive pain relief.

For those patients struggling with depression, pharmacogenetics may give the opportunity for the pharmacist to guide the provider to antidepressant medications with a greater chance for therapeutic effect and avoid failures that may take weeks to be evident. For example, a candidate patient is admitted with depression. The provider has chosen citalopram and the pharmacist has listed as the drug–gene pathway that citalopram uses as CYP2C19 extensive metabolizer and also SLC6A4 poor responder. When the SLC6A4 serotonin transporter is impaired, the phenotype increases the risk of citalopram failure by 2-fold and also increases the risk of adverse drug reactions for all selective SSRIs.[8,9] In other words, the likelihood of success with citalopram and other SSRIs is low. After reviewing the patient's other metabolic pathways, the pharmacist collaborating with the provider could suggest other antidepressants that are not SSRIs without known metabolic gene–drug pathway impairment (**Table 2**).

Medication Therapy Management and the Wellness Pharmacy

MTM is medical care provided by pharmacists whose goals are to customize drug therapy, incorporate personalized medicine, and improve therapeutic outcomes for patients. Wellness pharmacy also includes additional care paradigms, including immunizations, general health, wellness, and disease prevention educational measures (**Fig. 3**). Working directly with patients, the MTM model can provide a medication review after an initial patient assessment, create a treatment plan, educate the patient, and monitor the medication outcome. MTM includes 5 elements: medication therapy review, personal medication record, medication-related action plan (MAP), intervention and/or referral, and documentation and follow-up.[14] A medication therapy review is a systematic process of collecting patient and medication-related information that occurs during the face-to-face, pharmacist–patient encounter. In addition, the medication therapy review assists in the identification and prioritization of medication-related problems. During the MTM encounter, the pharmacist develops a personal medication record to be used by the patient. The personal medication record includes

Table 2
Combinatorial interpretation of pharmacokinetics and pharmacodynamics genetic results for an SSRI

Drug	Interaction Severity	Comments
Celexa (citalopram)		CYP2C19 ultrarapid metabolizer, increased metabolic clearance expected, with possible increased dose requirement. However, SLC6A4 poor responder phenotype indicates an increased risk of subtherapeutic response and side effects to SSRIs, thus a citalopram dose increase may not be effective. If clinically indicated, consider switch to non-SSRI that is not dependent on CYP2C19 ultrarapid metabolism or CYP2D6 poor metabolism such as desvenlafaxine, bupropion, or levomilnacipran.

An example interpretation for a patient taking citalopram who is found to be a CYP2C19 ultrarapid metabolizer and an SLC6A4 poor responder.
Abbreviations: CYP, cytochrome P; SSRI, selective serotonin receptor inhibitor.

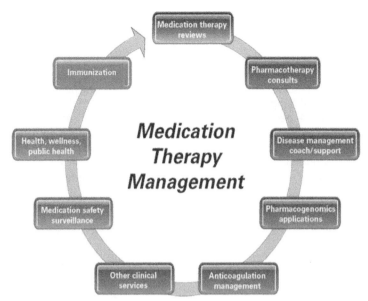

Fig. 3. Medication therapy management (MTM) processes. (Diagram recreated based on an original graphic developed by the American Pharmacists Association (APhA). Used with permission granted from APhA, July 2016.)

all prescription and nonprescription medications and requires updating and reviewing as needed. After assessing and identifying medication-related problems, the pharmacist develops a patient-specific MAP. The MAP is a list of self-management actions necessary to achieve the patient's specific health goals. In addition, the patient and pharmacist use the MAP to record actions and track progress toward health goals. During the MTM session, the pharmacist identifies medication-related problem(s) and determines appropriate intervention(s) for resolution. Often, the pharmacist collaborates with other health care professionals to resolve the identified problem(s). After the patient encounter and/or intervention, the pharmacist must document his or her encounter and determine appropriate patient follow-up.[14]

Currently, the pharmacist has access to the patient's current and past medications, current and past laboratory values and has an updated drug–drug interaction profile. Pharmacogenomics adds another source of information to personalize the medications to enhance outcomes, minimize adverse drug interactions, and avoid medication failure. We can illustrate how genetic information can enhance and give possible predictability for positive outcomes with the anticoagulation management of warfarin.

Traditional warfarin treatment currently incorporates the close monitoring of warfarin upon initiation of therapy by the MTM pharmacist. An overlap with unfractionated or low-molecular-weight heparin is required the first 5 days and until the international normalized ratio (INR) has reached therapeutic goal for 2 consecutive days. Warfarin antithrombotic effect is not achieved for at least 5 days and complete anticoagulation can take 10 or more days to achieve the goal INR. The patient may be scheduled for the first follow-up appointment 3 days after starting warfarin and depending on the INR have follow-up visits weekly or more frequently depending on those INR values. The dosing variability can be personalized by monitoring the INR response to specific doses.[15] The INR results can have wide variability from patient to patient with some achieving goal INR in 3 to 7 days and up to 42 days for others.[16] Two genetic tools that add predictability to warfarin are VKORC1 (the PD target, which reflects dose requirement) and CYP2C9 (the PK pathway, which reflects dose and time to steady state).[16–19]

The decreased expression of the VKOR enzyme owing to the VKORC1 -1639 G > A variant results in decreased warfarin demand to maintain anticoagulation. Patients with the low warfarin sensitivity genotype VKORC1 GG have the highest average daily dose requirements (4.5 mg) to maintain an INR between 2.0 to 3.0 in comparison with the intermediate GA genotype (3.8 mg) daily and the high sensitivity AA group (2.2 mg)[20] (**Fig. 4**). CYP2C9 variants, on the other hand, allow the pharmacist to estimate genetically where the patient may be in reaching a steady state for the INR. A patient with the normal CYP2C9*1/*1 genotype would have an estimated time to steady state of 3 to 5 days, CYP2C9*1/*2 has an estimated time to steady state of

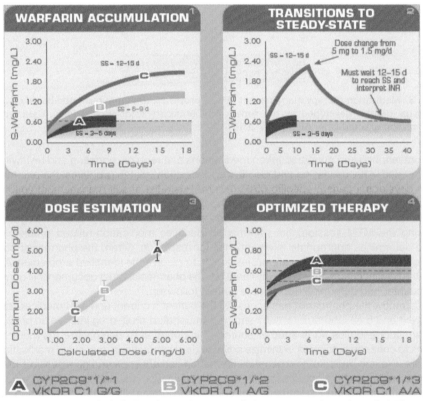

Fig. 4. Genotype-guided dosing for optimum warfarin concentrations. (*Panel 1*) Time to steady state (SS) and peak warfarin concentrations depend on the cytochrome P (CYP)2C9 genotype. (*Panel 2*) The transition to a new SS concentration after a dose adjustment depends on the half-life of the CYP2C9 variant; the international normalized ratio should be interpreted in the context of SS warfarin concentrations. (*Panel 3*) Algorithm-based maintenance dose estimates allow the physician to determine what optimal dose is required for each of 3 patients with the same physical characteristics but differing genotypes. (*Panel 4*) Genotype-based maintenance dose estimates facilitate optimized therapy, with the goal of every patient safely reaching the therapeutic range with the optimal effective dose to achieve stable anticoagulation. (*From* Reynolds KK, Valdes Jr R, Ramey-Hartung B, et al. Individualizing warfarin therapy. Pers Med 2007;4(1):24; with permission.)

6 to 9 days, and CYP2C9*3 is 12 to 15 days (see **Fig. 4**). Optimal interpretation of the INR and dose decisions based on that measurement are optimal when the INR is stable, meaning that it is representative of warfarin blood concentrations that have reached steady state. Once the blood concentrations are no longer transitioning upward, as would be the case upon initiation or dose escalation, then the INR can be trusted to be truly reflective of stability.[16]

Fig. 5 shows an actual patient who was initiated on warfarin 5 mg/d without pharmacogenetic testing with an INR goal between 2.0 and 3.0. The solid blue line indicates modeled blood concentrations that were accumulating as a consequence of the dosing regimen and the patient's CYP2C9 genotype; however, these concentrations were not known to the provider at the time; the only INRs, represented by gold boxes, were known measurements as per standard practice. The patient took 5 mg/d for 6 days, with low INRs on days 0 and 3. By the sixth day, the INR was 4.0 and the doses was held for 5 more days. By the return visit on day 11, the INR had fallen too low to 1.6. The patient as reinitiated on altering doses of 2 mg/d and 3 mg/d. Over the next week, the patient was more closely followed and exhibited 3 INRs in the therapeutic range. With those 3 measurements, the patient was considered stable on that dose and was not seen for another 10 days. By the next visit on day 31, the INR had spiked to 4.4 with no other clinical changes. The dose was again held for 2 days, at which point the INR decreased to 3.0. The dose was again held another 3 days, which resulted in another subtherapeutic INR of 1.5. On day 36, the dose was reinitiated at 2 mg/d and not until roughly 50 days after initiation was the patient finally stabilized in the therapeutic range. The patient was genotyped after stabilization and was found to carry the CYP2C9*2/*2 genotype, which predicts decreased clearance, decreased half-life, and therefore, a delay in the time to reach steady state. This patient did not reach steady state until 2 weeks after each dose change. In that window between days 15 and 22, when the 3 INR measurement were in the therapeutic range, that was an unfortunate "honeymoon" phase. They were therapeutic but not stable; the blood concentrations were still accumulating, albeit more slowly than anticipated because the genotype was not known. That is why the INRs were slow to react, not until steady state was achieved on day 31, 2 weeks after the dose change, had the

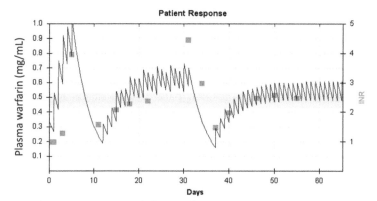

Fig. 5. Example patient genotyped for warfarin after initiation of therapy. *Blue lines* represent warfarin blood concentrations modeled after actual prescribed doses based on patient's cytochrome P (CYP)2C9 *2/*2 genotype-guided half-life. Gold boxes represent patient's actual measured international normalized ratios (INRs). The treating provider only knew the INRs and doses at the time of treatment. Blood concentrations demonstrate the effect genotype has on half-life and delayed to reach steady state.

blood concentrations finally stopped increasing, was then the true stabilization phase. The pharmacogenetic results for the patient also included a maintenance dose estimate based on the patient's age, gender, weight, target INR, and CYP2C9 and VKORC1 genotypes, which was estimated to be 2.2 mg/d.[20] The patient was stabilized on 2 mg/d but it took nearly 2 months. Use of the genetic results at initiation could have saved more than a month of trial and error dosing, during which time the patient was at risk of both thromboses as well as bleeding events owing to the multiple out of range INRs.

This example illustrates several critical concepts. "Therapeutic" and "stable" are not the same thing, they are not actually interchangeable pharmacologic properties. "Therapeutic" refers to the INR in the target range for the patient's indication, for example, 2.0 to 3.0. Pharmacologically, this implies nothing about stability of the blood concentrations, whether they are still transitioning (before 5 half-lives have been reached) or have plateaued. An INR can be in the therapeutic range yet still moving, as in the case example. "Stable" refers to the blood concentrations—and the INR as their surrogate marker—as having reached the steady-state plateau. Pharmacologically, this implies nothing about whether the stable blood concentrations (and stable INR) are actually within the therapeutic range. Indeed, they could be "stable" and very far outside of the therapeutic goal. CYP2C9 genotyping allows the MTM clinic pharmacist to estimate significant delays in the time to reach steady state for up to 40% of the population to better interpret each INR in the context of transitional versus stable drug levels. One should not infer for the patient with a 14-day time to reach steady state that INR measurements should wait 14 days to be measured, it means that all INRs measured per standard of care between days 0 to 14 should be interpreted as still transitioning, and interpreted with more caution. An INR on day 7 would only have transitioned half way to its final level, so if on day 7 it has already reached 2.5, the dose should probably be adjusted lower on that day to avoid the very likely supratherapeutic INR 1 week later. If, however, on day 7 the INR is still less than 2.0, waiting on a dose escalation may be the better decision to give the levels a chance to complete the increase. An inadvertent misinterpretation of the INR on day 7 as stable could lead to a premature dose increase and eventual supratherapeutic INR by day 14.

The pharmacogenetic paradigm shift is not to change the frequency of INRs, it is to interpret them more accurately as a reflection of the patient's true drug burden. When an INR is measured, the first question should no longer be "is it therapeutic" because therapeutic does not mean stable. The first question should be, "Is the patient likely to have reached steady state?" or in other words, "Have the drug levels plateaued?" and then second, ask "is it in the therapeutic range?" This shift affords the pharmacist the ability to decrease ADRs, decrease clinic visits owing to out-of-range patients, thereby increasing available time for new patients, and ultimately improves MTM clinic care.

SUMMARY AND FUTURE PERSPECTIVES

The future for pharmacogenetics in the context of pharmacy will continue to expand. Pharmacists have the chance to apply and incorporate drug knowledge in collaboration with physicians and other health providers using pharmacogenetics. This will not be just in a general broad context, but will be personalized for each patient reflecting that patient's drug–gene metabolic pathway. Patients with this personal approach benefit with enhanced therapeutic outcomes that potentially could lead to more streamlined drug approaches, fewer follow-up visits, cost savings, and shorter times to achieve therapeutic outcomes. In all pharmacy settings, having drug–gene metabolic pathways listed on the patient's electronic medical record and linked to medications similar to the system now used for allergies will allow the providers and pharmacists to avoid potential drug failures, customize initial doses and schedules, alert for multiple drugs using the same metabolic pathway, and prevent duplication therapies for medications that would be unlikely to provide therapeutic response. The time will arrive when, as in allergies/ADRs, no medication order can be processed without the knowledge of the patient's drug–gene metabolic pathway. This information and insight can substantially reduce ADRs and patient mortality. The clinical pharmacist placed inside a clinical laboratory now could have the unique opportunity to take laboratory results that were once posted in a static environment; waiting for action upon being viewed by the provider and now can make those laboratory results actionable and collaborate with the provider to improve medication outcomes in real time. In addition to a list of current medications and allergies, patients could carry a card listing their drug–gene metabolic pathways that they would present to their physicians and their pharmacists, potentially preventing medication misadventures. These drug–gene metabolic pathways could also be available as an application (phone app) on their mobile devices. As more drug–gene pathways are discovered and use of this knowledge increases, the potential for algorithm development for medication use will occur, resulting in better patient outcomes, higher standard of care, and reflect evidence-based medicine.

REFERENCES

1. Lazarou J, Pomeranz BH, Corey PN. Incidence of adverse drug reactions in hospitalized patients: a meta-analysis of prospective studies. JAMA 1998;279: 1200–5.
2. Pirmohamed M, James S, Meakin S, et al. Adverse drug reactions as cause of admission to hospital: prospective analysis of 18 820 patients. BMJ 2004;329:15–9.
3. Swen JJ, Nijenhuis M, de Boer A, et al. Pharmacogenetics: from bench to byte–an update of guidelines. Clin Pharmacol Ther 2011;89:662–73.
4. Crews KR, Gaedigk A, Dunnenberger HM, et al. Clinical Pharmacogenetics Implementation Consortium (CPIC) guidelines for codeine therapy in the context of cytochrome P450 2D6 (CYP2D6) genotype. Clin Pharmacol Ther 2012;91:321–6.
5. Crews KR, Gaedigk A, Dunnenberger HM, et al. Clinical Pharmacogenetics Implementation Consortium guidelines for cytochrome P450 2D6 genotype and codeine therapy: 2014 update. Clin Pharmacol Ther 2014;95:376–82.
6. Reynolds KK, Ramey-Hartung B, Jortani SA. The value of CYP2D6 and OPRM1 pharmacogenetic testing for opioid therapy. Clin Lab Med 2008;28:581–98.
7. Food and Drug Administration (FDA). FDA drug safety communication: safety review update of codeine use in children; new Boxed Warning and Contraindication on use after tonsillectomy and/or adenoidectomy. 2013. Available at: www.fda.gov/Drugs/DrugSafety/ucm339112.htm. Accessed June 17, 2016.
8. Kato M, Serretti A. Review and meta-analysis of antidepressant pharmacogenetic findings in major depressive disorder. Mol Psychiatry 2010;15:473–500.
9. Serretti A, Kato M, De Ronchi D, et al. Meta-analysis of serotonin transporter gene promoter polymorphism (5-HTTLPR) association with selective serotonin reuptake inhibitor efficacy in depressed patients. Mol Psychiatry 2007;12:247–57.
10. Zhang JP, Lencz T, Malhotra AK. D2 receptor genetic variation and clinical response to antipsychotic drug treatment: a meta-analysis. Am J Psychiatry 2010;167:763–72.

11. Hicks JK, Bishop JR, Sangkuhl K, et al. Clinical pharmacogenetics implementation consortium (CPIC) guideline for CYP2D6 and CYP2C19 genotypes and dosing of selective serotonin reuptake inhibitors. Clin Pharmacol Ther 2015;98:127–34.
12. Food and Drug Administration (FDA). Table of pharmacogenomic biomarkers in drug labeling. 2015. Available at: www.fda.gov/Drugs/ScienceResearch/ResearchAreas/Pharmacogenetics/ucm083378.htm. Accessed June 17, 2016.
13. Reyes-Gibby CC, Shete S, Rakvåg T, et al. Exploring joint effects of genes and the clinical efficacy of morphine for cancer pain: OPRM1 and COMT gene. Pain 2007;130:25–30.
14. American Pharmacists Association, National Association of Chain Drug Stores Foundation. Medication therapy management in pharmacy practice: core elements of an MTM service model (version 2.0). J Am Pharm Assoc 2008;48(3): 341–53.
15. Ansell J, Hirsh J, Hylek E, et al. Pharmacology and management of the vitamin K antagonists: American College of Chest Physicians evidence-based clinical practice guidelines (8th edition). Chest 2008;133:160S–98S.
16. Reynolds KK, Valdes R Jr, Ramey-Hartung B, et al. Individualizing warfarin therapy. Per Med 2007;4:11–31.
17. Bon Homme M, Reynolds KK, Valdes R Jr, et al. Dynamic pharmacogenetic models in anticoagulation therapy. Clin Lab Med 2008;28:539–52.
18. Borgman MP, Pendleton RC, McMillin GA, et al. Prospective pilot trial of PerMIT versus standard anticoagulation service management of patients initiating oral anticoagulation. Thromb Haemost 2012;108:561–9.
19. Hill CE, Duncan A. Overview of pharmacogenetics in anticoagulation therapy. Clin Lab Med 2008;28:513–24.
20. Zhu Y, Shennan M, Reynolds KK, et al. Estimation of warfarin maintenance dose based on VKORC1 (-1639 G>A) and CYP2C9 genotypes. Clin Chem 2007;53: 1199–205.

The Future of Precision Medicine in Oncology

Lori M. Millner, PhD, NRCC[a,b], Lindsay N. Strotman, PhD[a,c,*]

KEYWORDS

- Liquid biopsy • Targeted therapy • Circulating tumor cell (CTC)
- Cell-free nucleic acid (cfNA) • Exosomes • Extracellular vesicle (EV)

KEY POINTS

- Precision medicine in oncology is focused on identifying therapies that are based on genetic characterization of a patient's tumor.
- One of the newest additions to the precision medicine arsenal is the liquid biopsy, which is based on circulating tumor cells (CTCs), cell-free nucleic acid (cfNA), and exosomes.
- Liquid biopsies allow longitudinal information regarding a patient's tumoral genotype to be obtained through peripheral blood draws and are less invasive than traditional tissue biopsies.

NEED FOR PRECISION MEDICINE IN ONCOLOGY

Precision medicine in oncology is focused on identifying which therapies will be most effective for each patient based on genetic characterization of their cancer. Traditional chemotherapy is cytotoxic and destroys all cells that are rapidly dividing. The foundation of precision medicine is targeted therapies, first developed in the late 1990s. Targeted therapies inhibit specific molecules involved in tumor growth and dissemination of cancer cells. Studies have also been performed to discover targets that predict effectiveness in radiation therapy. The proportion of clinical trials requiring a genetic alteration for enrollment has increased dramatically over the past several years, and many studies have demonstrated benefit of targeted therapies over cytotoxic therapies in both progression-free survival (PFS) and overall survival (OS).[1,2]

Precision medicine requires an understanding of the vast heterogeneity and complexity of tumors as well as the processes that drive heterogeneity. Mechanisms of tumoral heterogeneity acquisition include somatic mutations, C > T transitions at CpG sites, activity of apolipoprotein B mRNA editing enzyme, therapy, chromothripsis,

Disclosure Statement: The authors have nothing to disclose.
[a] PGXL Technologies, 201 East Jefferson Street, Suite 306, Louisville, KY 40202, USA;
[b] Department of Pathology and Laboratory Medicine, University of Louisville, Louisville, KY, USA; [c] Department of Engineering, University of Louisville, Louisville, Kentucky, USA
* Corresponding author. PGXL Technologies, 201 East Jefferson Street, Suite 306, Louisville, KY 40202.
E-mail address: lindsay.strotman@pgxlab.com

and whole-genome doublings.[3] The result of these processes is a diverse tumor that can harbor many different subclonal populations. Currently, targeted therapies are often effective against only a subclonal population of cells; therefore, other methods that can better assess heterogeneity are needed. This review discusses roles that biomarkers serve, including predictive, prognostic, pharmacodynamic, and diagnostic purposes. The discussion includes targeted therapies already in use for many cancers as well as biomarkers in development. Special attention is paid to the rise of the use of liquid biopsies in the field of precision medicine in oncology, including CTCs, circulating cfNA, and extracellular vesicles (EVs).

TYPES OF BIOMARKERS: DIAGNOSTIC, PREDICTIVE, PROGNOSTIC, AND PHARMACODYNAMIC

"A biomarker is a characteristic that is objectively measured and evaluated as an indicator of normal biological processes, pathologic processes, or biological responses to a therapeutic intervention is the definition given by the Biomarkers Working Group."[4] This biomarker should serve as a sign of a normal or abnormal process or of a condition or disease.[5] The Food and Drug Administration (FDA) defines biomarkers into 4 general categories, mainly related to uses in therapy development. Several biomarkers can fall within multiple categories, because the surrogate endpoint can vary (**Fig. 1**).

1. Diagnostic biomarker: categorizes patients by presence or absence of a specific physiologic or pathophysiological state or disease
2. Prognostic biomarker: indicates degree of risk for disease occurrence or progression, distinguishing "good" and "poor" outcomes
3. Predictive biomarker: categorizes patients by the likelihood of response to a particular beneficial or harmful therapy

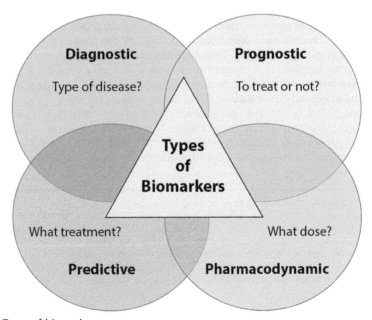

Fig. 1. Types of biomarkers.

4. Pharmacodynamic biomarker: shows a biological response has occurred to therapy prior to or after treatment; can be considered treatment-specific or informative of disease response

Due to the substantial risk of adversely affecting public health if a biomarker is falsely accepted as a surrogate endpoint, robust scientific evidence is needed to justify qualification of a biomarker before validation can even begin. Therefore, FDA-cleared assays using a biomarker in cancer have been limited.

FOOD AND DRUG ADMINISTRATION–CLEARED TESTS VERSUS LABORATORY DEVELOPED TESTS

In this discussion, tests that have been cleared by the FDA (FDA) and laboratory developed tests (LDTs) are included; however, there are distinctions between them. An LDT is a type of in vitro diagnostic test that is designed, manufactured, and used within a single laboratory. LDTs currently are not required to go through premarket review and other stringent requirements of FDA-cleared tests because they were considered simple tests.[6] Due to an increase of LDT use and complexity, on September 30, 2014, the FDA presented a new draft guidance to congress indicating increased FDA oversight of LDTs. The landscape is currently changing and laboratories must stay up to date regarding these changes and how they may affect the approval process of tests developed by laboratories.

The major types of cancer and how precision medicine is having an impact both on biomarker identification and treatment are examined. This discussion is not meant to be an exhaustive list of all cancer subtypes but, rather, examples of how precision medicine is influencing each discipline.

PRECISION MEDICINE IN BREAST CANCER

Breast cancer (BCa) is the most commonly diagnosed cancer for women both in the United States and globally. BCa is the second ranking cancer responsible for female mortality in the United States, causing an estimated 40,730 deaths in 2015.[7,8] The major types of targeted therapy in BCa include endocrine therapy, anti-HER2 therapy, PI3K, BRCA1/2, and CK4/6 inhibitors (**Table 1**). Some of the first targeted agents in oncology were developed against hormone receptor (estrogen receptor and

Table 1
Targeted therapies in breast cancer

Therapy	Drug	Type
Endocrine therapy	Tamoxifen	Selective estrogen receptor modulator
	Anastrozole	Aromatase inhibitor
	Exemestane	Aromatase inhibitor
	Letrozole	Aromatase inhibitor
	Fulvestrant	Estrogen receptor down-regulator
HER2 therapy	Trastuzumab	Monoclonal antibody
	Ado-trastuzumab emtansine	Antibody conjugated to cytotoxic agent (T-DM1)
	Lapatinib	Small molecule inhibitor
	Pertuzumab	Monoclonal antibody
CDK4/6 inhibitors	Palbociclib	Small molecule inhibitor
PI3K-mTOR inhibitors	Everolimus	Small molecule inhibitor

progesterone receptor)–positive BCa. Estrogen-focused therapies have remained part of the standard of care for more than 30 years. Tamoxifen modulates the estrogen receptor[9] and aromatase inhibitors decrease amount of estrogen produced,[10] whereas other agents, like fulvestrant, degrade the estrogen receptor.[11]

DIAGNOSTIC, PROGNOSTIC, OR PREDICTIVE TESTS

There are several prognostic and predictive assays using breast tumor tissue. Some of the most well-known predictive assays are Oncotype DX (Genomic Health, Redwood City, CA), MammaPrint (Agendia, Uíge, Angola), and Prosigna PAM50 (NanoString Technologies, Seattle, WA) and have been recently reviewed.[12] Likely the most well-known prognostic assay is the Oncotype DX, which uses reverse transcriptase (RT)–polymerase chain reaction (RT-PCR) to analyze expression of 16 cancer-related genes and 5 housekeeping genes. An algorithm analyzing expression of these genes generates a recurrence score that indicates which patients will benefit most from chemotherapy in addition to hormone therapy.[13] Both the American Society of Clinical Oncology (ASCO) and the National Comprehensive Cancer Network (NCCN) guidelines include Oncotype DX testing in their recommendations for estrogen receptor–positive, HER2-negative, and node-negative patients.[14] An FDA-cleared prognostic assay, MammaPrint, is included in some international recommendations.[15] This assay is based on microarray analysis of a 70-gene signature used to accurately select early-stage BCa patients who are highly likely to develop distant metastases and would benefit the most from adjuvant chemotherapy.[16] The Prosigna PAM50 is another FDA-cleared prognostic assay that uses RT-PCR to examine 50 genes identifying BCa subtypes. The PAM50 also determines a risk of recurrence score to determine prognosis and add significant information to commonly available immunohistochemistry markers.[17]

FDA-cleared tests
1. MammaPrint
2. Prosigna PAM50
3. GeneSearch BLN Test Kit (Janssen Diagnostics, Raritan, NJ): detects spread of BCa to lymph nodes by measuring 2 gene targets abundant in BCa tissue and scarce in lymph nodes
4. HER2 fluorescence in situ hybridization (FISH) assays
   a. INFORM HER2 Dual ISH DNA Probe Cocktail (Ventana, Oro Valley, AZ)
   b. *HER2* CISH pharmDxTM Kit (DAKO, Carpinteria, CA)
   c. Dako TOP2A FISH pharmDx Kit (DAKO, Carpinteria, CA)
   d. DakoCytomation Her2 FISH pharmDx Kit (DAKO, Carpinteria, CA)

LDTs
1. Oncotype DX
2. Genomic Grade Index (MapQuant Dx, Ipsogen, Marseille, France)
3. Breast Cancer Index (BioTheranostics, San Diego, CA)
4. EndoPredict (Sividon Diagnostics, Köln, Germany)

PRECISION MEDICINE IN NON–SMALL CELL LUNG CANCER

Lung cancer is the leading cause of cancer mortality. Lung cancer can be divided into small cell lung cancer (10%–15%) and non–small cell lung cancer (NSCLC) (85%).[8] The main NSCLC predictive biomarkers found in NSCLC include ALK fusion oncogene (anaplastic lymphoma kinase) and sensitizing epidermal growth factor receptor (EGFR) mutation. Currently, there are 3 FDA-cleared companion biomarker assays used to detect these biomarkers that are associated with different targeted therapies (**Table 2**). Other targeted therapies that have arisen include angiogenesis inhibitors and immune checkpoint inhibitors (see **Table 2**); however, there are currently no associated biomarkers.

DIAGNOSTIC, PROGNOSTIC, OR PREDICTIVE TESTS

Other emerging biomarkers in NSCLC as listed in the 2016 NCCN guidelines include KRAS, HER2, and BRAF V600E mutations; ROS1 and RET gene arrangements; MET amplification; and MET exon skipping mutation. For example, KRAS mutations can serve as a prognostic biomarker indicative of patient survival independent of treatment received[18] and as a predictive biomarker showing lack of therapeutic efficacy to EGFR targeted therapies.[19] Although FDA-cleared KRAS mutational detection assays have been approved for use in colorectal cancer (ie, cobas KRAS Mutation Test [Roche, Basel, Switzerland] and *therascreen* KRAS RGQ PCR Kit [Qiagen, Hilden, Germany]), they have not yet been approved for use in NSCLC. Additionally, the multiple biomarkers discovered in NSCLC have led to the development of mutational screening assays designed to detect multiple biomarkers simultaneously. Although a majority of these assays are usually performed using multiplex PCR, next-generation sequencing (NGS) panels have rapidly begun to appear, because both mutations and gene rearrangements can be detected simultaneously. No matter the detection scheme, the 2016 NSCLC NCCN guidelines are strongly endorsing use of these multiplexed assays.

FDA cleared
1. *therascreen* EGFR RGQ PCR Kit: a real-time PCR test for the qualitative detection of exon 19 deletions and exon 21 substitutions mutations in EFGR using DNA derived from formalin-fixed paraffin-embedded tumor tissue; received approval with gefitinib
2. cobas EGFR Mutation Test: a companion diagnostic for mutations in EGFR using DNA derived from formalin-fixed paraffin-embedded tumor tissue; received approval with osimertinib
3. Vysis ALK Break Apart FISH Probe Kit (Abbott Molecular, Santa Clara, California)

Table 2 Targeted therapies in non–small cell lung cancer		
Therapy	**Drug**	**Type**
Angiogenesis inhibitors	Bevacizumab	Monoclonal antibody targets VEGF-A
	Ramucirumab	Recombinant humanized monoclonal antibody targets VEGFR2
Tyrosine kinase inhibitors	Gefitinib	Small molecule EGFR inhibitor
	Erlotinib	Small molecule EGFR inhibitor
	Afatinib	Small molecule irreversible covalent EGFR and HER2 inhibitor
	Osimertinib	EGFR inhibitor
	Cetuximab	EGFR inhibitor
	Crizotinib	Small molecule ALK, ROS1, and MET inhibitor
	Ceritinib	Small molecule ALK and IGF-1 inhibitor
	Alectinib	Small molecule ALK and RET inhibitor
Immune checkpoint inhibitor	Nivolumab	Monoclonal antibody acting as immunomodulatory blocking PD-1 ligand activation on activated T cells
	Pembrolizumab	Humanized antibody to target PD-1

LDTs
1. Sequenom MassARRAY System (Agena Biosciences, San Diego, CA): a nonfluorescent detection platform using mass spectrometry to accurately measure PCR-derived amplicons. They have also developed the LungCarta® and LungFusion™ panel.
2. SnaPshot Multiplex System (Thermo Fisher Scientific, Waltham, MA): uses a primer extension-based method to multiplex up to 10 SNPS and detects using capillary electrophoresis
3. NGS or massively parallel sequencing
   a. Sentosa SQ NSCLC panel (VELA Diagnostics, Kendall, Singapore)
   b. Pervenio Lung NGS (Thermo Fisher Scientific): uses Ion AmpliSeq Lung Cancer Research Panel. Thermo Fisher also offers RNA Fusion Lung Cancer Research Panel.
   c. Lung Cancer Comprehensive Mutation and Translocation Panel (ARUP Laboratories, Salt Lake City, UT)
   d. Lung Cancer Mutation Panel (Quest Diagnostics, Madison, NJ)

PRECISION MEDICINE IN PROSTATE CANCER

Prostate cancer (PCa) is the most common solid tumor in men in the United States, ranking 5th in mortality and more than 230,00 cases diagnosed each year.[20] The main historical PCa biomarker is prostate-specific antigen (PSA). PSA screening has, however, garnered criticism over the years due to the possibility of overdetection, which has led to efforts to find other improved biomarkers.[7,12,21] The majority of effort in PCa biomarker development is to distinguish PCa from benign prostatic conditions with better sensitivity and specificity than PSA and to differentiate aggressive from nonaggressive PCa. Although there are currently 3 FDA-cleared tests and several other LDTs, new predictive and pharmacodynamic biomarkers are being pursued due to the development of targeted PCa therapies (**Table 3**). The main target of these therapies is the androgen receptor (AR), which is a main driver of PCa.[22]

DIAGNOSTIC, PROGNOSTIC, OR PREDICTIVE TESTS

FDA-cleared tests
1. Prostate Health Index (Beckman Coulter, Brea, CA; in partnership with the National Cancer Institute Early Detection Research Network): measures 3 forms of PSA to better distinguish PCa from benign prostatic conditions

Table 3
Targeted therapies in prostate cancer

Therapy	Drug	Type
Androgen synthesis inhibitors	Abiraterone acetate	Small molecule CYP17 inhibitor
	Ketoconazole	Small molecule CYP450 inhibitor
Antiandrogen	Enzalutamide	Small molecule AR inhibitor
	Flutamide	Small molecule AR inhibitor
	Bicalutamide	Small molecule AR inhibitor
	Nilutamide	Small molecule AR inhibitor
Immunotherapeutic	Sipuleucel-T	Autologous Cancer Vaccine

2. Prosensa (Gen-Probe, San Diego, CA): nucleic acid amplification test measuring PCa antigen 3 expression in urine to better distinguish PCa from benign prostatic conditions
3. CELLSEARCH Circulating Tumor Cell Kit (Janssen Diagnostics)

LDTs
1. Oncotype DX: measures expression of 12 cancer-related genes from small formalin-fixed paraffin-embedded tissue samples to discriminate PCa patients into very low, low, or intermediate risk groups that should be under active surveillance
2. Prolaris Score (Myriad Genetics, Salt Lake City, UT): measures tumor cells growth characteristics and expression of 46 different genes from prostate biopsy core specimens to stratify disease risk of progression
3. Prostarix (performed at Metabolon and offered by Bostwick Laboratories, Glen Allen, VA): measures signature of 4 metabolites from urine samples post–digital rectal examination using liquid chromatography–mass spectrophotometry
4. Mi-Prostate Score (University of Michigan Health System, Ann Arbor, MI): combines urine test for PCa antigen 3 from Progensa, TMPRSS2:ERG fusion, and serum PSA levels to produce risk assessment of PCa and aggressiveness
5. ConfirMDx (MDxHealth, Irvine, CA): detects an epigenetic specific profile (ie, DNA methylation) in prostate biopsy core specimens
6. Prostate Core Mitomic Test (MDNA Life Sciences, West Palm Beach, FL): detects mitochondrial DNA deletions in prostate biopsy core specimens
7. 4Kscore Test (Opko Lab, Nashville, TN): combines free PSA and total PSA, human kallikrein 2, and intact PSA measurements and considers age, digital rectal examination results, and prior biopsy status to determine the percent likelihood of finding high-grade cancer on biopsy

PRECISION MEDICINE IN MELANOMA

Rates of melanoma have risen faster than any other cancer over the past 2 decades with 75,000 new cases diagnosed each year.[23] These figures are thought to be underestimated, because many superficial and in situ melanomas treated in outpatient setting are not reported.[24]

Unlike other cancers, melanoma does not respond to chemotherapy or radiation, which has led to the development of immune and targeted therapies (**Table 4**). Approximately 50% to 60% of patients with metastatic melanoma have an activating mutation in V600 of BRAF (serine/threonine-protein kinase B-raf), an intracellular signaling kinase.[25] Although patients initially respond to BRAF inhibitors with increased PFS and OS, resistance usually arises due to alternative activation of other downstream targets in the same signaling kinase pathway. Therefore, other inhibitors

Table 4
Targeted therapies in melanoma

Therapy	Drug	Type
BRAF V600E inhibitors	Dabrafenib	Small molecule inhibitor
	Vemurafenib	Small molecule inhibitor
Immune checkpoint inhibitor	Ipilimumab	Monoclonal antibody
	Trametinib	Small molecule inhibitor
Tyrosine kinase inhibitor	Imatinib	Monoclonal antibody

(ie, MEK1 and MEK2) have been developed for downstream MAPK signal transduction pathways targets. Finally, immunotherapeutic agents have been developed that target immune checkpoint inhibitors, which harness the individual's own immune system to target and destroy cancerous cells.[26,27] These immune and targeted therapies are also summarized in **Table 4**.

DIAGNOSTIC, PROGNOSTIC, OR PREDICTIVE TESTS

Other kinase inhibitors are also being developed against additional mutations found in Melanoma as listed in the 2016 NCCN guidelines, including BRAF, NRAS, c-kit, GNA11 and GNAQ. KIT is the most notable example because there is already an FDA-cleared tyrosine kinase inhibitor used against Bcr-Abl in chronic myelogenous leukemia and gastrointestinal stromal tumors harboring a KIT mutation. A phase II study of 43 patients with KIT-mutated metastatic melanomas demonstrated a 23% overall response rate with this therapy, although response was of limited duration.[28] Finally, 10% of melanomas are attributed to hereditary predisposition resulting in the development of LDTs to identify individuals at risk, which is important for implementing strategies to reduce the burden of early disease.

FDA cleared
1. cobas® 4800 BRAF V600 (Roche): a companion diagnostic for V600 that received approval with BRAF inhibitor vemurafenib
2. THxID-BRAF (bioMèrieux, Marcy-l'Étoile, France): a companion diagnostic for V600E or V600K that received approval with BRAF inhibitors dabrafenib and trametinib

LDTs
1. myPATH (Myriad): measures expression of 23 different genes from melanoma lesions
2. NGS (includes only melanoma targeted panels performed in clinical laboratories and is only a brief, not comprehensive view of all the current panels available)
   a. IVD Sentosa SQ Melanoma Panel (Vela Diagnostics)
   b. Melanoma NGS Panel (Fulgent Diagnostics, Temple City, CA)
   c. Melanoma Targeted Gene Panel by NGS (Mayo Medical Laboratories, Rochester, MN)
   d. Hereditary Melanoma Panel (Baylor Miraca Genetics Laboratories, Houston, TX)
   e. Melanoma Hereditary Cancer Panel (ARUP Laboratories)

PRECISION MEDICINE IN COLORECTAL CANCERS

Colorectal cancer is the third most common cancer in both men and women, with an estimated 49,190 expected US deaths in 2016.[29] Much effort has been put into targeted therapies and diagnostic tests for this disease. Three main classes of targeted therapies have been approved to treat metastatic colorectal cancer, including multikinase inhibitors, angiogenic inhibitors, and anti-EGFR antibodies. These therapies are summarized in **Table 5**. Multikinase inhibitors include regorafenib, dabrafenib, and vemurafenib. Targets of regorafenib include angiogenic (VEGF1–3 and TIE2), stromal (PDGFR-β and FGF1), and oncogenic (KIT, RET, and B-RAF) protein kinases.[1,30] Clinical trials have demonstrated a modest increase in OS for patients on regorafenib. Dabrafenib and vemurafenib both inhibit the V600E mutation in BRAF, which is mutated in up to 15% of colorectal cancer cases and signifies poor prognosis.[31] Angiogenic inhibitors include bevacizumab and aflibercept. Bevacizumab inhibits vascular endothelial growth factor (VEGF), which plays a central role in the tumor

Table 5
Targeted therapies in colorectal cancer

Therapy	Drug	Type
Angiogenesis inhibitors	Bevacizumab	Monoclonal antibody – targets VEGF
	Aflibercept	Fusion protein – targets VEGF
Anti-EGFR therapy	Panitumumab	Monoclonal antibody
	Cetuximab	Monoclonal antibody
Multikinase inhibitors	Regorafenib	Small molecule inhibitor – angiogenic and oncogenic protein kinases
	Dabrafenib	Small molecule BRAF V600E inhibitor
	Vemurafenib	Small molecule BRAF V600E inhibitor

angiogenic pathway. When used in combination with chemotherapy, bevacizumab was shown to increase PFS and OS.[32] Aflibercept also targets VEGF and has demonstrated increased OS and PFS when used in combination with FOLFIRI.[29] EGFR signaling results in cell proliferation and migration. Anti-EGFR monoclonal antibodies include cetuximab and panitumumab. Studies have demonstrated that patients with nonmutated KRAS have increased PFS and OS when treated with either cetuximab or panitumumab in combination with FOLFIRI or FOLFOX compared with chemotherapy alone.[5,7,8]

DIAGNOSTIC, PROGNOSTIC, OR PREDICTIVE TESTS

In April of 2015, the American Society for Clinical Pathology, College of American Pathologists, Association for Molecular Pathology, and American Society for Clinical Oncology released a new set of recommendations and consensus opinions in anticipation of new guidelines for the Evaluation of Molecular Markers for Colorectal Cancer. The consensus guidelines strongly recommend RAS mutational testing for patients who are being considered for anti-EGFR therapy, KRAS, and NRAS (codons 12, 13 of exon 2; 59, 61 of exon 3; and 117 and 146 of exon 4). They also recommend BRAF V600 and deficient mismatch repair/microsatellite instability testing.

FDA-cleared tests
1. *therascreen* KRAS RGQ PCR Kit (Qiagen): a qualitative real-time PCR assay for the detection of specific mutations in the KRAS oncogene
2. cobas KRAS Mutation Test (Roche): PCR-based diagnostic test intended for the detection of mutations in codons 12 and 13 of the KRAS gene to select appropriate patients for treatment with cetuximab or panitumumab
3. Cologuard (Exact Sciences, Marlborough, MA): collects stool and examines elevated levels of altered DNA and/or hemoglobin associated with cancer/precancerous lesions

LDTs
1. KRAS Mutation Detection Kit (Trimgen, Sparks Glencoe, MD): based on a shifted termination assay andused to help select patients for panitumumab and cetuximab
2. ColoVantage (Quest Diagnostics): a blood test that detects methylated Septin9 DNA, which is a proved marker for colorectal cancer. This test is associated with an overall 70% sensitivity and 89% specificity.
3. Colox (Novogenix, Los Angeles, CA): measures the gene expression profile of 29 biomarkers by real-time PCR in peripheral blood mononuclear cells and uses an algorithm to diagnose colorectal cancer in a noninvasive manner

INTRODUCTION TO LIQUID BIOPSIES

A new precision medicine strategy in the field of oncology is the liquid biopsy. The use of liquid biopsies allows physicians increased longitudinal access to genetic material, providing greater opportunity for biomarker detection. Traditionally, tissue from a tumor is evaluated for malignancy using dyes, microscopes, and highly trained pathologists. Some tissue micrographs yield equivocal results due to poor staining or poor sample selection. In most cases, surgeons have only a single opportunity to obtain tissue from a patient. Liquid biopsy materials include CTCs, cfNA or EVs that are derived from primary and metastatic tumors and allow physicians access to longitudinal time points of a patient's disease (**Fig. 2**). This is accomplished because liquid biopsies are obtained from a peripheral blood draw that is much less invasive to the patient than traditional tumor tissue biopsies. The first commercial liquid biopsy test was offered in 2000, the CELLSEARCH. The CELLSEARCH assay enumerates CTCs that are known to be predictive in several epithelial cancer types. In recent years, the liquid biopsy field has matured beyond CTCs to include cfNA and EVs. cfNA typically constitutes a very small portion of a person's total circulating nucleic acids but can be useful for monitoring tumoral genetic variations. EVs, on the other hand, encapsulate nucleic acids, providing a protected environment, thus providing better stability specifically of RNA. This discussion provides information on CTCs, cfNA, and EVs for use as liquid biopsies.

CIRCULATING TUMOR CELLS

CTCs are cells that have been shed from a tumor and may be capable of forming metastases. Metastasis is the most dangerous and deadly facet of cancer and is responsible for 90% of cancer related deaths.[33] The metastatic process is accomplished by a CTC successfully carrying out a series of processes. First, the CTC must detach from the primary tumor and intravasate into the blood stream (see **Fig. 2**). Once in circulation, the CTC must survive a journey in the blood stream and extravasate into microvessels of a distant tissue. It must then adapt and survive in the microenvironment of the distant tissue. Finally, the CTC must colonize to form a metastatic lesion. The CELLSEARCH system for detection of CTCs is the only FDA-cleared assay for CTCs and is used as a predictor of OS and PFS in metastatic BCa patients. This method is based on detection of the epithelial markers, epithelial cell adhesion marker (EpCAM) and cytokeratins. Using this technology, however, CTCs are not detected in

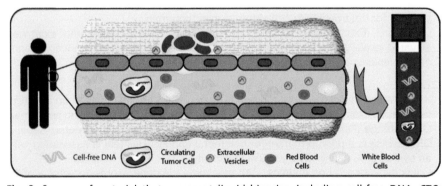

Fig. 2. Sources of material that represent liquid biopsies, including cell-free DNA, CTCs, and EVs.

40% of patients with metastatic BCa.[34–36] There are several other non–FDA-cleared methods for enumerating or isolating CTCs.[37] The methods for enriching or isolating CTCs include size-based isolation, nucleic acid–based detection, magnetic-activated cell separation (MACS), microfluidic-based isolation, and immunomagnetic isolation. These methods and companies pursuing them are listed in **Table 6**.

CELL-FREE NUCLEIC ACIDS

cfNAs circulating in blood were first described by Mandel and Metais in 1948[38]; however, it was not until 1994 when NRAS gene fragments were detected in cancer patients' blood, that the scientific community recognized cfNA's potential importance.[39,40] Since then, cfNA has become an essential tool in the liquid biopsy arsenal, gaining popularity over CTCs because cfNA isolation is deemed easier to obtain. cfNA is hypothesized to be released passively during apoptotic or necrotic events, with macrophages unable to clean-up the cell debris due to overproduction.[41] The average cfNA fragment is 180 to 200 base pairs, the same length that is released during cell death.[42] Secretion by cancer cells is also suggested as a mechanism of cfNA release. cfNA half-life is approximately 2 hours and levels have been reported to decrease dramatically after tumor removal and increase again if metastasis occurs.[43] The sensitivity and specificity of cfNA rely on the detection of common somatic alterations found in cancers. But cfNA's main limitation in cancer is that cfNA may not necessarily reflect physiologic and pathologic processes but can be associated in patients with tissue trauma, inflammatory disease, and so forth.[43] Benefits of cfNA include increased access to tumor heterogeneity compared to traditional tissue biopsy that often results in sample bias due to

Table 6
Methods for circulating tumor cell isolation

Method	Principle for Detection	Vendor
AdnaTest	RT-PCR of tumor-related transcripts	AdnaGen
ApoStream	Microfluidic-dielectric and morphology-based	ApoCell
Ariol	Immunodetection of cytokeratins 8, 18, and 19	Leica Microsystems
Biocept blood test	Microfluidic-biotinylated antibody capture	Biocept (San Diego, California)
BioFluidica CTC system	Microfluidic-antibody or aptamer capture	BioFluidica
CELLSEARCH	Immunodetection of cytokeratins 8, 18, and 19 with flow cytometry	Janssen Diagnostics
CTC-iChip	Microfluidic immunocapture	Janssen Diagnostics/Massachusetts General Hospital
CytoTrack CT11	Automated imaging	CytoTrack
DEPArray	Dielectrophoresis	Silicon Biosystems
Ikoniscope imaging system	Magnetic antigen expression	Ikonisys
ISET	Immunodetection of EpCAM	Rarecells
Parsortix	Microfluidic-size and deformability selection	Angle

spatial constraints. Lastly, liquid biopsies may be able to detect a tumor before it can be seen by imaging.

One challenge with cfNA compared with other types of liquid biopsy, is a background noise–to-signal problem requiring sensitive technologies. To this end, several investigators have pursued digital PCR technologies, which have a sensitivity of approximately 0.01% (ie, 1 mutated allele in presence of 10,000 wild-type alleles) or less.[44] Digital PCR differs from conventional in that the sample is divided into single molecules before amplification and detection, enabling more accurate quantification. The most notable companies are Raindance Technologies and Bio-Rad, which use droplet-based digital PCR by performing the PCR reactions in individual oil-water emulsion droplets. Life Technologies foregoes droplets, instead relying on thousands of nanofluidic wells to separate individual biomolecules. Targeted NGS represents the other sensitive technology being pursued; however, it is still a burgeoning technology because workflows are laborious and expensive. Additionally, bioinformatics teams are developing new algorithms to help with the signal-to-noise problem and ensure the signal is real (**Table 7**).

Table 7
Companies using cell-free nucleic acid to perform biomarker interrogation

Method	Principle for Detection	Vendor
Multiplex PCR, MassARRAY detection	Capture mutant amplicons on magnetic beads and detect by mass spec	Agena Biosciences (San Diego, CA)
Repetitive transient hybridization in alternating current field	Can detect 100 mutations down to 0.01% allelic frequency	Boreal Genomics (Vancouver, BC Canada)
Digital PCR	—	Chronix Biomedical (San Jose, CA)
Various PCR, NGS	Oncotype Seq Liquid Select	Genomic Health (Redwood City, CA)
NGS	Sequencing of ctDNA	Grail (Redwood City, CA)
Digital sequencing (PCR, barcoding, NGS)	LDTs cover 54 relevant oncogenes. Former Illumina research and development managers	Guardant Health (Redwood City, CA)
Tagged amplicon sequencing (Tam-Seq)	Identification of rare cancer mutations using NGS	Inivata (Research Triangle Park, NC)
Various PCR methods and NGS	Offer a wide variety of liquid biopsy services	MolecularMD (Cambridge, MA)
Multiplex PCR and NGS	Noninvasive prenatal test	Natera (San Carlos, CA)
PCR and NGS	Recently introduced METDetect-R plasma test	Personal Genome Diagnostics (Baltimore, MD)
Beads, emulsion, amplification, and magnetics (BEAMing) and NGS	Circulating tumor DNA allelic frequency 0.02%	Sysmex Inostics (Baltimore, MD)
Digital droplet PCR and NGS	Determine mutations in KRAS and BRAF from circulating tumor DNA; developing EGFR, NRAS, and PIK3CA	Trovagene (San Diego, CA)

EXTRACELLULAR VESICLES

EVs are the newest and least developed of liquid biopsy sources. EVs are membranous structures released by cells to the external environment. Their main function is intercellular communication, serving as vehicles to transfer cell of origin specific proteins, lipids, and nucleic acids between cells.[45] EVs can be distinguished into 4 categories mainly based on their size, cell origin, and secretion mechanisms. This nomenclature is still hotly debated (see Strotman LN, Linder M: Extracellular Vesicles Move Towards Use in Clinical Laboratories, in this issue) and in flux because tools to isolate the specific EV populations have not been developed.[46]

The traditional EV isolation method is ultracentrifugation, but it is laborious and time consuming and requires expensive instrumentation that is not amenable to most clinical laboratories. Therefore, new EV isolation methods are being developed. Although still in their infancy, these methods are being marketed as commercial kits for research and development. These kits are based on EVs' physical properties and include affinity chromatography, size exclusion chromatography, and precipitation.[47] Characterization of isolated EV is currently performed using biochemical analysis (ie, ELISA or Western blots), mass spectrophotometry, and various imaging techniques.[48] The main markers used in biochemical analysis include a 4 transmembrane domain family, tetraspanins (CD63, CD81, CD82, CD53, and CD37).[48]

Most assays being developed use mass spectrophotometry as the downstream analysis; however, nucleic acid based assays are rapidly becoming available because their sensitivity improves (ie, digital PCR and NGS). But the main advantage of EVs over other liquid biopsies types is that entrapped biomolecules seem to remain more stable because they are protected from ubiquitous RNases, avoiding issues of shipping and sample handling. Additionally, it has been shown that EVs serve as reservoirs containing enriched material specific to origin cell. Despite limited EV biology knowledge, clinical assays are rapidly being developed around EVs (**Table 8**). Exosome Diagnostics is at the forefront, having established collaboration and distribution agreements with Eli Lilly and Qiagen. Additionally, in 2015 and 2016 they plan to launch 2 LDT tests, for PCa—ExoIntelliScore Prostate—and for NSCLC—ExoDx *Lung*(ALK). They are also in the initial stages of trying to achieve FDA regulatory approval.

FUTURE OF PRECISION MEDICINE IN ONCOLOGY

The idea of using liquid biopsies is appealing due to several limitations of tissue biopsies:

- Biopsies are invasive and not practical for monitoring progression and recurrence overtime.

Table 8
Companies using extracellular vesicles to perform biomarker interrogation

Method	Principle for Detection	Vendor
Exosome extraction, RNA mutational analysis	Exosome extraction, RNA mutational analysis	Exosome Diagnostics (Cambridge, MA)
Enzyme-linked lectin-specific assay (ELLSA)	ELLSA	Exosome Sciences (Monmouth Junction, NJ)
ELISA for capture and assay	ELISA for capture and assay	HansaBioMed OU (Tallinn, Estonia)
Exosome extraction	Exosome extraction	System Biosciences (Palo Alto, CA)

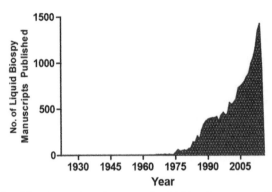

Fig. 3. Number of publications using the term, *liquid biopsies,* as quantified on PubMed.

- Tumor sample size can be limited due to its size and location, limiting the molecular testing that can be done.
- Cancer is a heterogeneous disease with molecular signatures that differ spatially and evolve over time as the disease progresses or due to therapy selective pressures.

These limitations drive the excitement behind liquid biopsies that include CTCs, cfNA, and EVs because they are cheaper, less laborious, and less invasive for the patient. The excitement is evident when examining the number of liquid biopsy publications which is increasing every year (**Fig. 3**).

With liquid biopsies, the stage can be set for diagnostic applications that include

- Early disease detection
- Monitoring treatment response and emerging molecular resistance
- Assessment of molecular heterogeneity and monitoring of tumor dynamics

To date the only FDA-cleared liquid biopsy platform is the CELLSEARCH system for CTC isolation, which serves as a prognostic indicator for breast, prostate, and colorectal cancer. Although CTCs are slightly ahead of the curve in technological development as a liquid biopsy, cfNA and EV are quickly catching up. For further liquid biopsy, however, implementation into clinical laboratories requires hurdles to be overcome including:

- Lack of standardization of sample collection, processing, and analysis
- Lack of large clinical trial validations

Although debate is focused heavily around the clinical utility of the different liquid biopsy samples, it is likely to remain until the field and technologies further mature. There is no reason to say, however, that the different types of liquid biopsy will not be complementary. For example, Exosome Diagnostics is using both cfNA and exosomes to increase the sensitivity of detecting EML4-ALK gene fusion in lung cancer patients. Cynvenio is also examining cfNA and CTCs simultaneously. As liquid biopsy sample preparation and detection become more robust and larger clinical trials are performed to prove clinical utility, it is likely that liquid biopsies will start to transform oncology treatment paradigms.

REFERENCES

1. Tobin NP, Foukakis T, De Petris L, et al. The importance of molecular markers for diagnosis and selection of targeted treatments in patients with cancer. J Intern Med 2015;278(6):545–70.

2. Roper N, Stensland KD, Hendricks R, et al. The landscape of precision cancer medicine clinical trials in the United States. Cancer Treat Rev 2015;41(5):385–90.

3. McGranahan N, Swanton C. Biological and therapeutic impact of intratumor heterogeneity in cancer evolution. Cancer Cell 2015;27(1):15–26.

4. Biomarkers Definitions Working Group. Biomarkers and surrogate endpoints: preferred definitions and conceptual framework. Clin Pharmacol Ther 2001; 69(3):89–95.

5. Sawyers CL. The cancer biomarker problem. Nature 2008;452(7187):548–52.

6. Administration, U.S.F.a.D. 2015. Available at: fda.gov. Accessed November 17, 2015.

7. Lee YJ, Park JE, Jeon BR, et al. Is prostate-specific antigen effective for population screening of prostate cancer? A systematic review. Ann Lab Med 2013;33(4): 233–41.

8. Siegel RL, Miller KD, Jemal A. Cancer statistics, 2015. CA Cancer J Clin 2015; 65(1):5–29.

9. Early Breast Cancer Trialists' Collaborative Group. Effects of chemotherapy and hormonal therapy for early breast cancer on recurrence and 15-year survival: an overview of the randomised trials. Lancet 2005;365(9472):1687–717.

10. Gibson L, Lawrence D, Dawson C, et al. Aromatase inhibitors for treatment of advanced breast cancer in postmenopausal women. Cochrane Database Syst Rev 2009;(4):CD003370.

11. Robertson JF, Llombart-Cussac A, Rolski J, et al. Activity of fulvestrant 500 mg versus anastrozole 1 mg as first-line treatment for advanced breast cancer: results from the FIRST study. J Clin Oncol 2009;27(27):4530–5.

12. Wong LM, Neal DE, Johnston RB, et al. International multicentre study examining selection criteria for active surveillance in men undergoing radical prostatectomy. Br J Cancer 2012;107(9):1467–73.

13. Paik S, Shak S, Tang G, et al. A multigene assay to predict recurrence of tamoxifen-treated, node-negative breast cancer. N Engl J Med 2004;351(27): 2817–26.

14. Lang JE, Wecsler JS, Press MF, et al. Molecular markers for breast cancer diagnosis, prognosis and targeted therapy. J Surg Oncol 2015;111(1):81–90.

15. Senkus E, Kyriakides S, Ohno S, et al. Primary breast cancer: ESMO Clinical Practice Guidelines for diagnosis, treatment and follow-up. Ann Oncol 2015; 26(Suppl 5):v8–30.

16. Mook S, Van't Veer LJ, Rutgers EJ, et al. Individualization of therapy using Mammaprint: from development to the MINDACT Trial. Cancer Genomics Proteomics 2007;4(3):147–55.

17. Wallden B, Storhoff J, Nielsen T, et al. Development and verification of the PAM50-based Prosigna breast cancer gene signature assay. BMC Med Genomics 2015; 8:54.

18. Slebos RJ, Kibbelaar RE, Dalesio O, et al. K-ras oncogene activation as a prognostic marker in adenocarcinoma of the lung. N Engl J Med 1990;323(9):561–5.

19. Eberhard DA, Johnson BE, Amler LC, et al. Mutations in the epidermal growth factor receptor and in KRAS are predictive and prognostic indicators in patients with non-small-cell lung cancer treated with chemotherapy alone and in combination with erlotinib. J Clin Oncol 2005;23(25):5900–9.

20. Sartori DA, Chan DW. Biomarkers in prostate cancer: what's new? Curr Opin Oncol 2014;26(3):259–64.

21. Vickers AJ, Lilja H. We need a better marker for prostate cancer. How about renaming PSA? Urology 2012;79(2):254–5.

22. Heinlein CA, Chang C. Androgen receptor in prostate cancer. Endocr Rev 2004;
    25(2):276–308.
23. Karagiannis P, Fittall M, Karagiannis SN. Evaluating biomarkers in melanoma.
    Front Oncol 2014;4:383.
24. Linos E, Swetter SM, Cockburn MG, et al. Increasing burden of melanoma in the
    United States. J Invest Dermatol 2009;129(7):1666–74.
25. Long GV, Menzies AM, Nagrial AM, et al. Prognostic and clinicopathologic asso-
    ciations of oncogenic BRAF in metastatic melanoma. J Clin Oncol 2011;29(10):
    1239–46.
26. Hodi FS, O'Day SJ, McDermott DF, et al. Improved survival with ipilimumab in pa-
    tients with metastatic melanoma. N Engl J Med 2010;363(8):711–23.
27. Robert C, Long GV, Brady B, et al. Nivolumab in previously untreated melanoma
    without BRAF mutation. N Engl J Med 2015;372(4):320–30.
28. Guo J, Si L, Kong Y, et al. Phase II, open-label, single-arm trial of imatinib mesy-
    late in patients with metastatic melanoma harboring c-Kit mutation or amplifica-
    tion. J Clin Oncol 2011;29(21):2904–9.
29. American Cancer Society. Cancer Facts & Figures 2015. Atlanta: American Can-
    cer Society; 2015. Available at: http://www.oralcancerfoundation.org/facts/pdf/
    Us_Cancer_Facts.pdf.
30. Wilhelm SM, Dumas J, Adnane L, et al. Regorafenib (BAY 73-4506): a new oral
    multikinase inhibitor of angiogenic, stromal and oncogenic receptor tyrosine ki-
    nases with potent preclinical antitumor activity. Int J Cancer 2011;129(1):245–55.
31. Safaee Ardekani G, Jafarnejad SM, Tan L, et al. The prognostic value of BRAF
    mutation in colorectal cancer and melanoma: a systematic review and meta-anal-
    ysis. PLoS One 2012;7(10):e47054.
32. Hurwitz H, Fehrenbacher L, Novotny W, et al. Bevacizumab plus irinotecan, fluo-
    rouracil, and leucovorin for metastatic colorectal cancer. N Engl J Med 2004;
    350(23):2335–42.
33. Fidler IJ. The pathogenesis of cancer metastasis: the 'seed and soil' hypothesis
    revisited. Nature reviews. Cancer 2003;3(6):453–8.
34. Cristofanilli M, Hayes DF, Budd GT, et al. Circulating tumor cells: a novel prog-
    nostic factor for newly diagnosed metastatic breast cancer. J Clin Oncol 2005;
    23(7):1420–30.
35. Witzig TE, Bossy B, Kimlinger T, et al. Detection of circulating cytokeratin-positive
    cells in the blood of breast cancer patients using immunomagnetic enrichment
    and digital microscopy. Clin Cancer Res 2002;8(5):1085–91.
36. Hayes DF, Cristofanilli M, Budd GT, et al. Circulating tumor cells at each follow-up
    time point during therapy of metastatic breast cancer patients predict
    progression-free and overall survival. Clin Cancer Res 2006;12(14 Pt 1):4218–24.
37. Millner LM, Linder MW, Valdes R Jr. Circulating tumor cells: a review of present
    methods and the need to identify heterogeneous phenotypes. Ann Clin Lab Sci
    2013;43(3):295–304.
38. Mandel P, Metais P. Les acides nucléiques du plasma sanguin chez l'homme. C R
    Seances Soc Biol Fil 1948;142(3–4):241–3 [Article in Undetermined Language].
39. Vasioukhin V, Anker P, Maurice P, et al. Point mutations of the N-ras gene in the
    blood plasma DNA of patients with myelodysplastic syndrome or acute myelog-
    enous leukaemia. Br J Haematol 1994;86(4):774–9.
40. Sorenson GD, Pribish DM, Valone FH, et al. Soluble normal and mutated DNA se-
    quences from single-copy genes in human blood. Cancer Epidemiol Biomarkers
    Prev 1994;3(1):67–71.

41. Schwarzenbach H, Hoon DS, Pantel K. Cell-free nucleic acids as biomarkers in cancer patients. Nat Rev Cancer 2011;11(6):426–37.
42. Jiang P, Chan CW, Chan KC, et al. Lengthening and shortening of plasma DNA in hepatocellular carcinoma patients. Proc Natl Acad Sci U S A 2015;112(11): E1317–25.
43. Diehl F, Schmidt K, Choti MA, et al. Circulating mutant DNA to assess tumor dynamics. Nat Med 2008;14(9):985–90.
44. Sausen M, Parpart S, Diaz LA Jr. Circulating tumor DNA moves further into the spotlight. Genome Med 2014;6(5):35.
45. Raposo G, Stoorvogel W. Extracellular vesicles: exosomes, microvesicles, and friends. J Cell Biol 2013;200(4):373–83.
46. Gould SJ, Raposo G. As we wait: coping with an imperfect nomenclature for extracellular vesicles. J Extracell Vesicles 2013;2.
47. Witwer KW, Buzás EI, Bemis LT, et al. Standardization of sample collection, isolation and analysis methods in extracellular vesicle research. J Extracell Vesicles 2013;2:20360.
48. Lotvall J, Hill AF, Hochberg F, et al. Minimal experimental requirements for definition of extracellular vesicles and their functions: a position statement from the International Society for Extracellular Vesicles. J Extracell Vesicles 2014;3:26913.

Understanding the Food and Drug Administration's Jurisdiction Over Laboratory-Developed Tests and Divisions Between Food, Drug, and Cosmetic Act–Regulated and Clinical Laboratory Improvement Amendments of 1988–Regulated Activities

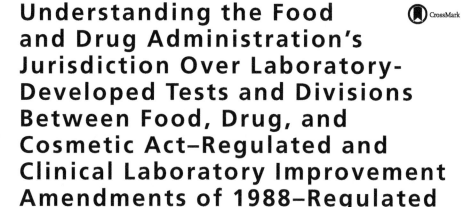

CrossMark

Bradley Merrill Thompson, MBA, JD, Bonnie I. Scott, JD,
James A. Boiani, MS, JD*

KEYWORDS

- LDT • IVD • Laboratory-developed test • FDA • Laboratory tests • CLIA

KEY POINTS

- The Food and Drug Administration has a strong case for its claims of jurisdiction over laboratory-developed tests under the Federal Food, Drug, and Cosmetic Act (FDCA).
- Developing a dividing line between regulation of laboratory-developed tests as articles under the FDCA and the analytical services provided by clinical laboratories under Clinical Laboratory Improvement Amendments of 1988 will pose a challenge to implementing an efficient and effective regulatory framework.
- Without a clear framework, any new regulatory system could be a major challenge to navigate, and could lead to duplicative regulation.

The scope of the Food and Drug Administration's (FDA's) jurisdiction over laboratory-developed tests (LDTs), and whether FDA has such jurisdiction at all, has been a heavily debated issue over the past several years. With FDA's release of draft guidance in October 2014 detailing its proposed framework for regulating many

Disclosure Statement: The authors represent both diagnostics companies and clinical laboratories who are impacted by potential regulation of laboratory-developed tests.
Epstein Becker & Green, PC, 1227 25th Street Northwest, Suite 700, Washington, DC 20037, USA
* Corresponding author.
E-mail address: jboiani@ebglaw.com

Clin Lab Med 36 (2016) 575–585
http://dx.doi.org/10.1016/j.cll.2016.05.005
0272-2712/16/$ – see front matter © 2016 Elsevier Inc. All rights reserved.
labmed.theclinics.com

LDTs,[1] the issue has become even more contentious. On a basic level, there are 2 sides to the debate: (1) those who believe FDA's efforts to expand its authority to regulate LDTs are unlawful and detrimental to the practice of medicine and diagnostic innovation; and (2) those who believe FDA should step in to regulate at least a subset of LDTs due to the potential harm they may cause in the absence of regulation. The former tend to include clinical laboratories and hospitals, whereas the latter tend to include FDA, certain patient groups, and in vitro diagnostics (IVD) manufacturers.

If FDA moves forward with its guidance, or Congress takes action to reform LDT and IVD regulation, a fundamental question that needs to be answered is how to divide activities regulated by the Food, Drug, and Cosmetic Act (FDCA) from those regulated by the Clinical Laboratory Improvement Amendments of 1988 (CLIA). Without a clear framework, any new regulatory system could be a major challenge to navigate, and could lead to duplicative regulation. Unfortunately, in the LDT debate, we rarely get to into these important details because both sides are entrenched in arguing generalities: FDA can do anything it wants or nothing at all with respect to LDTs. Therefore, in this article, we consider FDA's authority to regulate LDTs and the policy implications of regulation, and discuss an idea for a fact-driven framework to distinguish FDCA and CLIA activities.

FRAMING THE LEGAL ISSUES

The FDCA gives FDA jurisdiction over devices in interstate commerce for commercial distribution. In the following few pages we consider 3 questions that frame the legal issues with respect to this jurisdictional trigger, and whether it allows FDA to reach LDTs and the laboratories that make them.

Are In Vitro Diagnostic Devices Defined Narrowly as Packaged Kits or Something Broader?

A common issue of dispute in the debate over FDA's authority is over the identity of in vitro diagnostics. Often, those who argue that FDA's reach does not extend to LDTs say that the agency's authority is limited to packaged kits that are sold to the laboratories. As a starting place, we therefore consider whether FDA's authority is limited to these test kits or are more extensive.

The statutory definition of a medical "device" under the FDCA is very broad, and gives FDA the authority to regulate instruments, in vitro reagents, and other similar or related articles "intended for use in the diagnosis of disease or other conditions, or in the cure, mitigation, treatment, or prevention of disease, in man...."[2] FDA has interpreted this statute as giving it authority over in vitro diagnostic devices, among other things. Under FDA's regulations, "In vitro *diagnostic products* are those reagents, instruments, and systems intended for use in diagnosis of disease or other conditions, including a determination of the state of health, in order to cure, mitigate, treat, or prevent disease or its sequelae. Such products are intended for use in the collection, preparation, and examination of specimens taken from the human body."[3]

Within the definition of "in vitro diagnostic devices," the terms "reagents" and "instruments" are straightforward, and refer to items used to conduct a laboratory test. However, the term "systems" is somewhat less tangible. This is because FDA regulates the collection of all those things used to conduct an in vitro diagnostic test, as specified in labeling. Therefore, the "system" is determined mostly off the written word, but to some extent based on features that reveal intent that 2 items be used together. The scope of the system is determined by the all-important "intended use" of the system.

In addition to considering each of the terms included in the "device" and "in vitro diagnostic device" definitions, it is also critical to consider what these definitions do not say. Significantly, such definitions do not include any mention of co-packaging, or of shrink-wrapped kits, or any other language that suggests that the products that together comprise the in vitro diagnostic must be together somehow in a box or "kit." Often the various elements of an in vitro diagnostic arrive in separate packages to a laboratory.

Based on the preceding, that FDA's authority under the FDCA is not limited to packaged kits, but extends broadly to include systems and other products that may be made by a laboratory.

Are Tests That Never Leave the Laboratory in Interstate Commerce for Commercial Distribution?

The US Constitution empowers the federal government to "regulate Commerce-...among the several states,"[4] and this Constitutional authority is what underlies the FDCA.[5] An LDT is not, however, transferred by a laboratory across state lines. Indeed, an LDT may never leave the room it is created in. Therefore, a natural question is whether an LDT, even if it is a device, falls within the extent of the FDCA?

The Supreme Court has not taken such a narrow reading. It is well-settled law that products that have a (1) a substantial effect on and (2) a nexus to interstate commerce are themselves in "interstate commerce"[6]; physical transport across state lines is not required. In light of the fact that (1) LDTs generate billions of dollar in revenue, and play a fundamental role in managing the diagnosis and treatment of disease across the country; (2) many laboratories advertise and promote their LDTs using instrumentalities of interstate commerce (eg, e-mail, Internet, roads), often across state lines, and receive samples throughout the United States; and (3) many LDTs are often constructed using components that were themselves in interstate commerce, it is hard to argue that LDTs would fall outside the scope of the FDCA.

LDTs are being introduced into interstate commerce for "commercial distribution." "Commercial distribution" is defined as "any distribution of a device intended for human use which is *held or offered for sale*."[7] Courts have found that a product is "held for sale," and in commercial distribution when it is used in providing a medical service, even if never sold (or intended to be sold) in a commercial sense. For example, a court concluded that an optometrist using (but not selling) various medical devices in treating his patients' ocular conditions was holding those devices for sale (thus placing them in "commercial distribution").[8]

Based on the preceding, most LDTs can be considered articles in interstate commerce for commercial distribution. Given that those articles also meet the definition of a device, it would appear that FDA has jurisdiction over those products.

Can Laboratories Ever Be Manufacturers?

Even if LDTs appear to be devices subject to FDA regulation, a common argument in the LDT debate is whether a clinical laboratory itself can be regulated by FDA as a manufacturer. The definitions of "device" and "in vitro diagnostic device" are agnostic as to who actually makes the article, but some people argue there is an exemption for clinical laboratories.

To be clear, there is no provision in the FDCA that provides such an exemption.[9] Also, the CLIA contains no exceptions that would limit the definition of in vitro diagnostic devices. Instead, some people argue that CLIA creates a singular regulatory framework for clinical laboratories that is insulated from the FDCA. This position has not been embraced by FDA, or by the Centers for Medicare and Medicaid Services

(CMS), which administers CLIA and which has stated that FDA and CLIA "regulatory schemes are different in focus, scope and purpose, but they are intended to be complementary,"[10] with the former regulating the diagnostics themselves and the latter regulating performance of test services.

However, it is helpful to explore this issue through some hypotheticals.

Assume that a clinical laboratory were to buy an existing IVD company (which manufactures FDA-regulated IVDs).[11] Would that acquisition alone change FDA's jurisdiction over the IVDs the manufacturer produces? There is nothing in the FDCA or CLIA that indicates it would. A change in shareholders has no impact on the FDA's jurisdiction over the products a company produces. This is equally true if the new shareholders are somehow engaged in the practice of medicine: if a doctor owns a medical device company, the medical devices produced are not enveloped in the practice of medicine simply because the doctor owns the company.

Building on that hypothetical, consider the following 3 questions. For ease of reference, the clinical laboratory will be referred to as "Bradley's ClinLab, Inc.," and the IVD company as "Thompson's IVD Co."

1. If Bradley's ClinLab, Inc. decides to tell Thompson's IVD Co. that it (Thompson's) may only sell to Bradley's, does the FDA lose jurisdiction over the IVD that Thompson's makes?

No. Contractually requiring Thompson's IVD Co. to only supply Bradley's ClinLab would not change the regulatory status of the IVDs that Thompson's IVD Co. makes. The regulatory status of an IVD is based on the intended use of the reagents and instrument systems in diagnosing patients, and does not change based on commercial agreements that might limit the number of companies that could purchase those products.

This question is quite realistic because Bradley's ClinLab may want to become the sole provider of clinical laboratory services that use the IVD manufactured by Thompson's. If Thompson's IVD is particularly innovative, Bradley's ClinLab can enhance the value it offers by being the sole supplier of laboratory services making use of Thompson's IVD. Thus, whatever diminished sales there might be of Thompson's IVD to other clinical laboratories might be offset by the increased sales to Bradley's ClinLab.

From the parent company standpoint (ie, Bradley's ClinLab), sales would go up substantially. Presumably, Bradley's would widely promote the availability of the exclusive laboratory testing service that makes use of the Thompson's IVD, basically wrapping the IVD product in a clinical laboratory service.

2. If Bradley's ClinLab, instead of buying Thompson's IVD Co., builds an IVD company to be the same as Thompson's IVD Co., does that change the FDA's jurisdiction over the IVDs that the homegrown company makes?

No. There is nothing in the law that would distinguish between buying an IVD company and building an IVD company for FDA jurisdiction purposes. The law is solely focused on activities related to making reagents and/or instruments intended for use in the diagnosis of disease or other conditions, not how those activities come to be.

The only fact changing from the prior hypothetical is moving from buying an IVD company to building an IVD company. So assume, for the sake of this hypothetical, that this is the only difference. The resulting company has all of the same people and processes. Bradley's ClinLab simply built the company instead of buying it.

3. If, rather than managing Thompson's IVD Co. as a separate company, Bradley's ClinLab decides to merge the IVD operations into Bradley's ClinLab, does that merger mean that the FDA loses the ability to regulate the IVD manufacturing?

No. Merging 2 corporations into 1, and moving from 2 different facilities into 1, does not change FDA's jurisdiction over the IVD operations. As already explained, it is the nature of the activities that determines FDA's jurisdiction.[12]

This hypothetical question focuses on corporate law distinctions between 2 companies, and the difference between an acquisition and a merger. This question contemplates a corporate merger instead of the corporate acquisition. There would be no change in the actual operations of the clinical laboratory or the IVD operations, except potentially that they might be housed under 1 roof at 1 location.

In conclusion, as the hypotheticals illustrate, there is nothing special about the fact that an entity involved in manufacture of an IVD is a clinical laboratory: it would be treated under law like any IVD manufacturer.

POLICY IMPLICATIONS

The answers to the preceding questions lead to the conclusion that FDA can regulate IVDs made at clinical laboratories; that is, LDTs, even if they never leave the laboratory bench. However, the inquiry should not end there. Another critical question is: what constitutes making an IVD at a clinical laboratory? More specifically, how do regulators tell the difference between making IVDs at a clinical laboratory and testing services performed in the laboratory under CLIA?

This determination is complicated because the tasks performed by clinical laboratory professionals conducting clinical laboratory services clearly overlap with, and indeed in some cases look identical to, IVD manufacturing operations. The following is a list of examples of activities that might be performed either by a technician at a clinical laboratory or a technician at an IVD manufacturing establishment:

- Making a mixture of 3 fluorescent markers that are coupled with different clusters of designation markers for use in immunophenotyping.
- Adding interference filters to the optical chamber of a flow cytometer to enhance signal quality.
- Installing custom sequencing data analysis software on a Next Generation Sequencing platform.
- Altering the pH of a buffer solution used in testing to enhance sample stability.
- Developing a process (system) for extracting certain analytes from blood samples using various pieces of equipment and reagents together.

If a regulator walked into a building and just saw one of those operations being performed, the regulator may not know if he or she was standing in a clinical laboratory or an IVD manufacturer's establishment. Therefore, what is needed is a method of differentiating the types of activities occurring in clinical laboratories, which really fit appropriately within the practice of laboratory medicine subject to CLIA oversight, from the types of activities occurring in clinical laboratories, which really fit appropriately in the IVD manufacturing category subject to FDA oversight. Developing such a method and clear rule is a difficult task, but it can be done.

The first step is to examine precedent. This is not the first time FDA has been tasked with determining when activities being conducted by some type of health care professional are part of the practice of medicine or cross the line into FDA jurisdiction. Consider, for example, the following FDA enforcement initiatives:

1. Drugs manufactured for or by physicians and administered to patients as a part of the physician's medical practice: In some ways, this is where FDA started approximately 100 years ago when medical professionals were making and marketing various elixirs to their patients.
2. Medical devices reprocessed by hospitals: To save money, rather than dispose of single-use medical devices, some hospitals chose to reprocess them. Yet, reprocessing a single-use medical device is treated the same under the law as manufacturing a new device. The fact that hospitals are the ones doing the reprocessing is of no consequence; FDA regulates the activity.[13] In these cases, the reprocessed devices are not being sold to patients, but rather used by doctors.
3. The promotion by ophthalmologists of medical procedures using Lasik technology: Over the past several years, FDA has become concerned that ophthalmologists using FDA-cleared laser technology are promoting the use of that technology without adequately disclosing to their patients the associated risks in promotional statements. It is important to recognize that in these cases, what the doctors are selling is the medical procedure that makes use of the device. FDA has been sending enforcement letters to doctors who downplay the risks of using this particular technology in this particular procedure.[14,15]

The fact that an individual practices medicine (ie, provides a medical service) has never by itself been a defense to a charge by FDA that the person is violating the FDCA. Instead, the issue is whether the activity involved better fits within the practice of medicine regulated by the state boards of medicine or the manufacturing of a drug or device regulated by FDA. Of course, this is not always an easy question to answer.

Additional precedent that may be instructive is FDA's regulation of pharmacy compounding activities. Although pharmacy compounding is very different from the performance of laboratory services (and the 2 types of services have very different risk profiles), from a legal perspective, they present similar issues. **Table 1** crosswalks the legal frameworks related to pharmacy compounding and LDTs.

Both cases, pharmacy compounding and LDTs, have highly educated health care professionals, who are trained to provide complex services and who are regulated under specialized regulatory programs.

The practice of compounding allows pharmacists to tailor drugs to unique patient needs that cannot be met by an FDA-approved medication. Patients who benefit from compounding include patients with rare diseases or allergies that require a drug to be made without a certain dye or who cannot tolerate certain dosage forms (eg, a child who cannot swallow a pill and needs the drug in liquid form). Pharmacists can lawfully compound drugs for these purposes. In fact, in these instances, pharmacy compounding is not just lawful; it is an extremely important practice that undoubtedly saves many lives. Compounding activities are regulated by state boards of pharmacy, just as the activities of clinical laboratory practice are regulated by CMS under CLIA. And just as with the practice of medicine more generally, because there is a specialized regulatory program in place, FDA does not regulate traditional compounding.

However, there comes a point when a compounding pharmacist could start behaving more like a drug manufacturer than a pharmacist. Simply because pharmacists are being regulated by state boards of pharmacy does not mean that anything the pharmacist does cannot be regulated by any other governmental agency. Consider the extreme example of a pharmacist who begins printing dollar bills. The US Secret Service would have no difficulty pursuing enforcement against the

Table 1
Comparative history of LDT and pharmacy compounding issues

	Pharmacy Compounding	LDTs
Historical practices FDA protects	Under traditional pharmacy practice, pharmacists have compounded drugs behind the drugstore counter, working with physicians to provide personalized treatments for individual patients.	Under the traditional practice of clinical laboratory testing, laboratories have sought to fill in the gaps in approved, commercially available tests. Those gaps exist because of the huge variety of diseases and conditions, many of which are unique.
Historical policy approach	Although FDA says all compounded products are subject to FDA regulation, the agency has historically exercised considerable discretion to enable pharmacies to continue this traditional type of pharmacy practice. FDA took this position, in part, because • There are state boards of pharmacy; and • The agency did not have the resources to regulate every customized drug provided by a corner pharmacy.	FDA has historically taken the position that it has the authority to regulate laboratory-made tests, but is exercising enforcement discretion to permit the practice to continue. The agency typically offers 2 reasons for this approach: • CLIA and comparable state-level laws regulate the practice of clinical laboratory testing; and • The agency did not have the resources to regulate every custom-made clinical laboratory test.
Change in the nature of the practice	Some pharmacies began to develop into large-scale "compounding" operations that are far removed from traditional compounding, promote their drugs as alternatives to FDA-approved products for the same uses, and look more like drug manufacturing activities.	Some clinical laboratories began to engage in large-scale making of tests with complex components, promote their tests as alternatives to FDA-approved tests for the same uses, and look more like diagnostic test manufacturing activities.
FDA's policy responses	In 1992, FDA issued its first Compliance Policy Guide providing criteria for distinguishing when a pharmacy crossed the line from traditional pharmacy practice into large-scale drug manufacturing subject to FDA regulation, including premarket approval.	In 2014, FDA issued its proposed framework for regulating certain types of LDTs.

Abbreviations: CLIA, Clinical Laboratory Improvement Amendments of 1988; FDA, Food and Drug Administration; LDT, laboratory-developed test.

pharmacist even though the pharmacist is regulated by the state board of pharmacy. As another example, if a pharmacist bought a drug manufacturing company, no one would seriously contend that the drug manufacturing company ceased to be regulated by FDA just because it is owned by a pharmacist. Simply put, the applicable law will turn on the particular activities in which a pharmacist engages.

So where exactly is the dividing line between (1) traditional compounding that is regulated under the state boards of pharmacy, and (2) compounding that crosses over into drug manufacturing that requires compliance with FDA rules? On its face, much like laboratory services and IVD manufacturing, the actual process of producing a drug looks remarkably the same whether done by a pharmacist or by a drug manufacturer.

To clarify the difference, FDA developed a Compliance Policy Guide that explained the factors FDA would weigh in determining whether a pharmacy had crossed the line into drug manufacturing.[16] The task was difficult enough that FDA could not provide a singular definition of "drug manufacturing," or specific "check boxes" a pharmacy could use to determine if it had crossed the line. Instead, FDA offered the following list of potential pharmacy activities that it would consider holistically, not mechanically, to determine whether a pharmacy's activities raised the same types of concerns associated with drug manufacturers:

1. Compounding of drugs in anticipation of receiving prescriptions, except in very limited quantities in relation to the amounts of drugs compounded after receiving valid prescriptions.
2. Compounding drugs that were withdrawn or removed from the market for safety reasons.
3. Compounding finished drugs from bulk active ingredients that are not components of FDA-approved drugs without an FDA-sanctioned investigational new drug application (IND).
4. Receiving, storing, or using drug substances without first obtaining written assurance from the supplier that each lot of the drug substance has been made in an FDA-registered facility.
5. Receiving, storing, or using drug components not guaranteed or otherwise determined to meet official compendia requirements.
6. Using commercial-scale manufacturing or testing equipment for compounding drug products.
7. Compounding drugs for third parties who resell to individual patients or offering compounded drug products at wholesale to other state-licensed persons or commercial entities for resale.
8. Compounding drug products that are commercially available in the marketplace or that are essentially copies of commercially available FDA-approved drug products. In certain circumstances, it may be appropriate for a pharmacist to compound a small quantity of a drug that is only slightly different from a FDA-approved drug that is commercially available. In these circumstances, FDA will consider whether there is documentation of the medical need for the particular variation of the compound for the particular patient.
9. Failing to operate in conformance with applicable state law regulating the practice of pharmacy.

According to FDA, this list is not intended to be exhaustive, and other factors may be appropriate for consideration in a particular case.

A FRAMEWORK FOR DIVIDING FOOD, DRUG, AND COSMETIC ACT–REGULATED FROM UNREGULATED ACTIVITIES

The pharmacy compounding analogy provides guidance as to how the line might be drawn between laboratory services regulated under CLIA, and IVD manufacturing that FDA regulates, even if both are conducted in a clinical laboratory. Although FDA has already identified many of these factors in its October 2014 draft guidance, certain additional criteria are worth noting. It helps to organize the criteria into 2 different buckets: (1) criteria that focus on the public health implications of LDTs, and (2) criteria that focus on the legal distinction between the practice of medicine and the practice of manufacturing.

Public Health Criteria

These are practical criteria that the agency applies to minimize public health risk or negative impact. Notably, in November 2015, FDA released a report detailing the public health evidence for FDA oversight of LDTs, which includes case studies that illustrate how LDTs may have or did cause harm in the absence of compliance with FDA requirements.[17] In adopting these public health criteria, FDA's goal is to regulate high-risk uses. Turning back to the pharmacy compounding analogy, these public health criteria are similar to the second item listed previously from the Compliance Policy Guide (ie, compounding drugs that were withdrawn or removed from the market for safety reasons).

Specifically, FDA proposes not to regulate LDTs (1) that are low risk, (2) intended for rare diseases, and (3) intended for unmet medical needs. FDA proposes not to regulate those applications because either they are low risk or because there is no other feasible way that patients with those needs would have access to the necessary tests.

Legal Criteria

In addition to the public health criteria, FDA should apply criteria that stem from the legal task at hand, separating those activities that Congress intended to regulate under CLIA from those activities that Congress intended to regulate under FDA's rules. These criteria are not so much risk-focused but rather focused on identifying the characteristics of IVD manufacturing. Based on the pharmacy compounding precedent, FDA could use the following kinds of factors:

1. Test materials are made in advance of receiving an order from a physician for the test, and stored until such time as a physician places an order.
2. Tests that duplicate already manufactured tests, with a similar narrow exception as described under pharmacy compounding for small batches of slight variants.
3. Test materials made using manufacturing equipment and manufacturing processes not customarily used in laboratory testing services (eg, a commercial-scale filling system to pre-make reagent cocktails for later use in the laboratory).
4. Promotion of the protocol as evidence that it is really the protocol that is being sold.[18]
5. Whether the LDT is designed and used by a single laboratory.
6. Whether the LDT is composed only of components and instruments that are legally marketed for clinical use (eg, analyte-specific reagents [21 C.F.R. § 864.4020], general purpose reagents [21 C.F.R. § 864.4010], and various classified instruments).
7. Whether the LDT is both manufactured and used by a health care facility laboratory (such as one located in a hospital or clinic) for a patient that is being diagnosed and/or treated at that same health care facility or within the facility's health care system.
8. Whether the LDT is interpreted by qualified laboratory professionals, without the use of automated instrumentation or software for interpretation.

Some of these criteria are not precisely stated, and that is part of the challenge. Judgment needs to be applied regarding the totality of the circumstances. However, if applied in good faith, these criteria would lead to a clear answer for many tests; tests that fall in a gray area might require dialogue between FDA and the laboratory.

SUMMARY

It appears that the following 2 extreme statements are equally untrue:

1. *FDA's position that it has the legal authority to regulate all LDTs*. This is not true, as some LDTs fall within the practice of medicine and are thereby excluded from FDA jurisdiction.
2. *The position of many laboratories that FDA has no legal authority to regulate any LDTs*. That is also not true. A primary fallacy here is in the argument that "laboratorians provide the service, therefore the service is part of the practice of medicine." A laboratorian could provide tax preparation services, but the tax services would hardly be part of the practice of medicine. The focus needs to be on the "what" (ie, the activities), not just the "who."

Understanding the scope of FDA jurisdiction, and in particular discerning the dividing line between the practice of laboratory medicine and IVD manufacturing, requires a much more nuanced analysis. It requires separating out those specific activities that Congress intended to regulate under CLIA from those specific activities that Congress intended to regulate under the FDCA. Careful consideration must be given to the language of CLIA and the FDCA, as well as the specific facts regarding what laboratories are actually doing in their laboratories.

REFERENCES

1. FDA, Draft guidance for industry, FDA staff, and clinical laboratories: framework for regulatory oversight of laboratory developed tests. 2014. Available at: http://www.fda.gov/downloads/MedicalDevices/DeviceRegulationandGuidance/GuidanceDocuments/UCM416685.pdf. Accessed February 5, 2016.
2. 21 U.S.C. § 321(h).
3. 21 C.F.R. § 809.3.
4. US Const. Art. I, § 8, cl. 3.
5. *See e.g.*, FDCA § 301 (prohibiting "[t]he introduction…into interstate commerce of any food, drug, device, tobacco product, or cosmetic that is adulterated or misbranded").
6. *See Gonzales v. Raich*, 545 U.S. 1, 17 (2005) ("Our case law firmly establishes Congress' power to regulate purely local activities that are part of an economic "class of activities" that have a substantial effect on interstate commerce.").
7. 21 CFR § 807.3(b) (emphasis added).
8. *United States v. DeviceLabeled Cameron Spitler Amblyosyntonizer*, 261 F. Supp. 243, 245 (D. Neb. 1966). Importantly, in explaining its rationale for its decision, the court said: "Although the claimant never sold the devices in the commercial sense, the device was used in the claimant's treatment of patients".
9. It is no accident that FDA ended up with the authority to regulate in vitro diagnostic devices. In the late 1960s, FDA struggled to develop a regulatory framework for in vitro diagnostics, and that struggle is a substantial part of what led to the 1976 Medical Device Amendments. Congress very consciously made the decision to give FDA the authority to regulate these collections of reagents and instruments, intended to be used together in conducting a laboratory test.

10. CMS, LDT, and CLIA FAQs. 2013. Available at: https://www.cms.gov/Regulations-and Guidance/Legislation/CLIA/Downloads/LDT-and-CLIA_FAQs.pdf. Accessed February 5, 2016.
11. This hypothetical represents a very legitimate business decision. Companies in many industries vertically integrate. In business terms, vertical integration simply means buying a supplier. Companies will vertically integrate to diversify and grow, but also to better control the supply of some key product, and to control the cost of that product.
12. Further, FDA law has long held that intercompany transfers can still qualify as being "held for sale" as that term is used in the FDCA. Being held for sale is one of the ways that a product intended for diagnostic use can be placed in "commercial distribution," which gives FDA jurisdiction over that product (device). FDA regulations provide that "[i]nternal or interplant transfer of a device between establishments within the same parent, subsidiary, and/or affiliate company" fall outside the definition of "commercial distribution." 21 C.F.R. § 807.3(b)(1). This exemption cannot save a transfer from one unregistered establishment to another unregistered establishment.
13. FDA, center for devices and radiological health, guidance for industry and for FDA Staff: enforcement priorities for single-use devices reprocessed by third parties and hospitals. 2000. Available at: http://www.fda.gov/downloads/Medical Devices/DeviceRegulationandGuidance/GuidanceDocuments/ucm107172.pdf. Accessed February 5, 2016.
14. FDA, FDA letter to eye care professionals. 2011. Available at: http://www.fda.gov/ MedicalDevices/ProductsandMedicalProcedures/SurgeryandLifeSupport/LASIK/ ucm272960.htm. Accessed February 5, 2016.
15. FDA, warning letter to 20/20 Institute, Indianapolis Lasik. 2012. Available at: http:// www.fda.gov/ICECI/EnforcementActions/WarningLetters/2012/ucm333453.htm. Accessed February 5, 2016.
16. FDA, Compliance Policy Guide (CPG), Sec. 460.200: Pharmacy Compounding (issued 1992; reissued 2002; withdrawn 2013). Available at: http://www.fda. gov/OHRMS/DOCKETS/98fr/02D-0242_gdl0001.pdf. Accessed February 5, 2016. This CPG was declared obsolete based on recent legislation surrounding pharmacy compounding, the Drug Quality and Security Act. 78 Fed. Reg. 72901 (Dec. 4, 2013).
17. FDA, the public health evidence for FDA oversight of laboratory developed tests: 20 case studies. 2015. Available at: http://www.fda.gov/downloads/AboutFDA/ ReportsManualsForms/Reports/UCM472777.pdf. Accessed February 5, 2016.
18. Using promotion in this context does not run afoul of the First Amendment analysis under the Supreme Court decision in Thompson v. Western States Medical Center, 535 U. S. 357. 2002. Here promotion plays the same role it does in intended use. It is simply looked at as a factor to determine what the laboratory actually intends to sell.

Extracellular Vesicles Move Toward Use in Clinical Laboratories

Lindsay N. Strotman, PhD[a,b,]*, Mark W. Linder, PhD, DABCC[a,c]

KEYWORDS

- Liquid biopsy • Oncology • Extracellular vesicle (EV)

KEY POINTS

- Extracellular vesicles (EVs) are membranous particles found in a variety of biofluids that encapsulate molecular information from the cell, from which they originate.
- This rich source of information that is easily obtained can then be mined to find diagnostic biomarkers.
- The biological function of EVs are still evolving, but include, intercellular communication, coagulation, inflammation, immune response modulations, waste management and disease progression.
- Interest in EVs has expanded but much still needs to be done for EVs to reach their full potential as a source material in laboratory developed tests for personalized medicine, especially in oncology.

INTRODUCTION

The research field of extracellular vesicles (EVs) has expanded exponentially, leading to rapid spread of use in clinical applications. EVs are membranelike particles released from cells into biological fluids, including but not limited to blood, breast milk, salvia, urine, and cerebral spinal fluid.[1,2] EVs were first recognized as "platelet dust" in experiments studying blood coagulation.[3–5] Concurrently, EVs were isolated from conditioned culture medium and termed "exosomes."[6] Since then, additional studies of EVs have shown they contain lipids, proteins, and nucleic acids, reflecting their cellular origin[7,8]; therefore, analysis of their content can provide a rich source of clinical information. The biological function of EVs is still evolving, but includes, intercellular communication, coagulation, inflammation, immune response modulations, waste management, and disease progression.[8–10]

The authors have nothing to disclose.
a PGXL Technologies, 201 East Jefferson Street, Suite 306, Louisville, KY 40202, USA; b Department of Engineering, University of Louisville, Louisville, Kentucky, USA; c Department of Pathology and Laboratory Medicine, University of Louisville School of Medicine, 511 S Floyd Street, MDR Building, Room 204, Louisville, KY 40292, USA
* Corresponding author. PGXL Technologies, 201 East Jefferson Street, Suite 306, Louisville, KY 40202.
E-mail address: lindsay.strotman@pgxlab.com

Clin Lab Med 36 (2016) 587–602
http://dx.doi.org/10.1016/j.cll.2016.05.004
0272-2712/16/$ – see front matter © 2016 Elsevier Inc. All rights reserved.

In this review, we discuss the current consensus on EV classifications, then give a basic overview of EV isolation methods, as well as common EV detection and characterization techniques. We also briefly explore promising EV-based diagnostic applications within the oncology field. Throughout this review, we discuss major problems facing the EV field, in addition to their advantages and disadvantages for clinical use.

CURRENT EXTRACELLULAR VESICLE NOMENCLATURE

EVs is a blanket term used to describe different types of vesicles released from cells.[8] Current nomenclature, although controversial, is based on EV size, biogenesis, and cellular release mechanisms[11] (**Fig. 1**). The best studied EV types are exosomes and microvesicles. Exosomes range in diameter from 30 to 100 nm. Exosomes originate from intracellular multivesicular bodies that fuse with and are secreted by the plasma membrane.[12–15] Microvesicles are also referred to interchangeably as ectosomes and have a larger diameter, ranging from 50 to 2000 nm. Microvesicles directly bud or shed from the plasma membrane.[16,17] Another EV type is apoptotic bodies, sometimes classified as a specialized type of microvesicle. Apoptotic bodies are released during apoptotic membrane blebbing that occurs during the late stages of programmed cell death. Apoptotic bodies have a large diameter, ranging in size from 1 to 4 μm.[18] A final specialized EV type, not recognized by all investigators, is large oncosomes. Large oncosomes range in diameter from 1 to 10 μm and to some they are a branch of microvesicles. Large oncosomes differ from other EV types based on their abundant oncogenic cargo and specialized release by tumor cells.[19,20] Unfortunately, current EV isolation methods cannot discriminate between different EV types, because specific EV physical and chemical biomarkers are still lacking. These differences and other differences in upstream sample preparation have made it difficult to interrupt clinical insights.

PREANALYTICAL SAMPLE PREPARATION CONSIDERATIONS

Currently, there is no standardization of preanalytical steps, including sample collection apparatus, blood collection tube type, centrifugation speeds, or sample storage.[2,21]

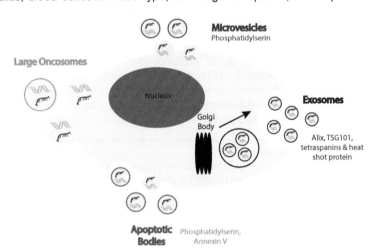

Fig. 1. Different types of extracellular vesicles and their biogenesis. Common protein identification markers for microvesicles, exosomes, and apoptotic bodies common protein markers are given.

However, standardization is needed to compare EV studies across different laboratories and elucidate the clinical usefulness of EVs. Unfortunately, standardization has been difficult owing to our incomplete understanding of how preanalytical sample preparation methods influences downstream results. The International Society for Extracellular Vesicles, International Society of Thrombosis and Hemostasis, and International Society for Extracellular Vesicles have had discussions on this subject and published some recommendations.[2,22–25] However, more preanalytical sample preparation comparison studies is needed to advise a complete set of recommendations. Below is a brief list of important preanalytical information that should be collected and current sample preparation advice surrounding the most common biofluid, blood.

- Patient details: age, sex, ethnicity, medications, fasting status, and medical history.
- Time sample collected.
- Larger needles for venipuncture should be used to avoid shear stress and prevent platelet activation, which causes further EV release.[26,27] Additionally, the first few milliliters of blood should be discarded to avoid fibroblast contamination.[28]
- Time of collection to centrifugation should be recorded because longer incubation times may result in higher EV counts.[29]
- Choice of anticoagulant (ie, blood tube type) is importance owing to its functional influence on EVs and downstream effect of analysis. For example, heparin is not suggested because it inhibits polymerase chain reactions (PCR).[30] Heparin has also been found to bind EVs, block EV uptake by cells, and lower the platelet activation threshold.[31,32] Anticoagulants based on calcium chelation are commonly used for EV analysis. Citrate tubes are preferred over ethylenediaminetetraacetic acid tubes, which have been shown to affect EV concentration.[33]
- Choice of serum or plasma as starting material for EV isolation. Plasma is preferred, because serum has been found to contain 50% more EVs, mainly associated with the blood coagulation process.[34]
- Centrifugation details (ie, rotor type, rcf, k-factor, and time) to separate plasma are highly variable. Most require an initial lower speed centrifugation to remove red blood cells and other circulating cells followed by a higher speed to remove platelets. Changes in viscosity should also be recorded, especially if using ultracentrifugation or density centrifugation for EV isolation.[35] Use of centrifugation can result in destruction or artificial creation of EVs, as well as EV aggregation.[21]
- Sample storage is commonly performed before analysis and for transportation. Although EVs have been shown to be more resistant to freeze/thaw cycles,[36,37] studies on effects on EV quantification have been limited.[33,38] Additionally, studies on how different types of EVs are effected is needed.

Unfortunately, preanalytical steps vary frequently depending on the research question or clinical study being conducted. Therefore, detailed preanalytical experimental variables should be included in publications as best outlined by Witwer and colleagues.[2] This also helps to establish future standardized preanalytical recommendation. Currently, as upstream preanalytical methods remain to be studied, the best advice is to try to keep these variables the same throughout a study.

EXTRACELLULAR VESICLE ISOLATION METHODS (ADVANTAGES AND DISADVANTAGES)

A robust method to isolate EVs would provide consistent measurements and minimize simultaneous isolation of contaminants, such as proteins and other membranous products. This is critical to identifying specific biologically relevant EV diagnostic biomarkers. Currently, EVs are isolated based on their physiochemical properties, including size, density, and surface composition. The traditional gold standard for EV isolation is ultracentrifugation, which is the most used method.[39] However other methods, such as ultracentrifugation, density gradient centrifugation, precipitation, size exclusion chromatography, affinity, and novel microfluidic techniques have emerged.[2] It should be noted that none of these individual EV isolation methods can isolate the different EV types; therefore, caution should be taken when designing and interpreting EV experiments.[40,41]

Ultracentrifugation

Ultracentrifugation forces vary in range for larger EVs from 10,000 to 20,000×g with smaller EVs pelleted at higher speeds ranging from 100,000 to 120,000×g. Ultracentrifugation times also vary widely, with 16 hours being traditional.[41] A disadvantage of ultracentrifugation is the requirement of specialized and expensive equipment. Additionally, sedimentation of contaminating protein complexes and lipoproteins occur owing to similar size and density.[35,42,43] Finally, aggregation of EVs is a common occurrence.[21] Attempts have been made to standardize ultrafiltration, but differences in upstream sample dilutions and rotors have made it more difficult.[44]

Density Gradient Centrifugation

To further reduce centrifugation speeds and contaminants, density gradient centrifugation (ie, sucrose or iodixanol) has gained popularity.[2,45] However, it should be noted that centrifugation times are longer than ultracentrifugation and vary from 62 to 90 hours.[46,47] It has also been reported that dilution of samples in an isosmotic solution before centrifugation increases the efficiency of EV isolation.[4,35] Contamination still occurs, because there are other things in blood with similar densities to EVs.

Polymer-Based Precipitation

In precipitation, a biofluid containing EVs is incubated with a polymer solution (ie, polyethylene glycol), usually overnight and then centrifuged at low speeds the next day. The part of the sample that pelletizes or "precipitates out" contains the EVs. Precipitation reagents are commercially available (ExoQuick [System Biosciences, Palo Alto, CA] and Total Exosome Isolation Kit [ThermoFisher Scientific, Waltham, MA]) and widely used owing to ease of handling.[48,49] However, demonstration of sample purity varies widely with some groups reporting superior purity to other EV isolation methods[50,51] and others low purity.[52] These differences are often a result of how investigators define purity.

Size Exclusion

EVs are separated based on their size differences by passage through or around physical barriers, such as a porous filters or chromatography resins. Commercially available kits are manufactured by qEV (Izon Sciences, Cambridge, MA) and ExoMir (Bioo Scientific, Austin, TX). These kits, as well as several investigators, use gravity to move fluids through the physical barriers, which helps to reduce forces on the sample that may result in EV deformation and aggregation.[53] Again results have been mixed concerning sample purity between different groups[42]; however, the EVs have been found to remain biologically active.[43,54,55]

Affinity

Isolation of EVs through affinity methods depends on specific EV surface proteins (antibody–antigen) or physiochemical properties. In affinity methods, the EVs bind to a solid phase resin, such as magnetic beads or columns, and the contaminants are washed away.[56–58] Although affinity affords highly specific EV isolation, prior EV biological knowledge must be available.[59] Additionally, EV yields are lower than other EV isolated methods.[60] Most affinity methods are homebrewed, but there are commercially available kits, including Immunobeads and ExoTEST (Hansa BioMed, Tallinn, Estonia), Dynabeads (ThermoFisher Scientific), and exoEasy (Qiagen, Hilden, Germany).[61]

Microfluidic

EV isolation microfluidic devices are being developed owing to their perceived cost effectiveness and potential for integration with multiple downstream analytical methods. Microfluidic devices currently published for EV isolation are based on affinity and size exclusion mechanisms.[62–64] Although initial published methods are promising, the input sample volume limits the yield of EVs isolated. In many cases, the EV yield is not compatible with downstream detection analytics.

EXTRACELLULAR VESICLE DETECTION AND CHARACTERIZATION METHODS

Multiple EV detection methods exist with no single method being able to simultaneously characterize EV size distribution, concentration, morphology, and biochemical composition. Therefore, detection methods are variable among investigators and often used in tandem. At present, the International Society for Extracellular Vesicles has published minimal experimental requirements for defining the detection of EVs.[65] A brief overview of common EV detection and characterization methods is presented, but this list is not meant to be exhaustive.

Focus on Morphology, Concentration, and Size Distribution Analysis

Electron microscopy

Scanning, transmission, and cryo electron microscopy are well-established methods for EV morphology, concentration, and biochemical analysis, but are low throughput and labor intensive. EM measures electrons and not photons, which have a longer wavelength, limiting its resolution.[24] EV biochemical composition is measured through the use of immunogold labeling.[66] However, because EVs require extra sample processing (ie, heavy metal stain, dehydration, and fixation), sample artifacts such as distorted size and shape can be introduced.[67] These problems can be mitigated by using cyro-EM, which does not dehydrate or chemically fix the sample.[1,68,69] Finally, size distribution and concentration determination is difficult owing to the limited number of EVs imaged.

Atomic force microscopy

Atomic force microscopy is akin to a record player, which uses a mechanical cantilever passed near the surface to measure deflection and create a 3-dimensional surface map. Atomic force microscopy has the best resolution (subnanometer), but can take hours to collect data depending on size of the area scanned.[66] Like EM, atomic force microscopy measures size distribution and morphology,[70,71] but is not recommended for determining concentration. Limited biochemical information can be obtained if EVs are captured by an antibody-coated surface before atomic force microscopy.[72]

Nanoparticle tracking analysis

Nanoparticle tracking analysis is a commercially available optical method that illuminates EVs with a laser beam so that light scatter can be detected. The light scatter allows individual EVs to be detected so that their mean velocity can be measured. Mean velocity is then plugged into Stokes-Einstein equation, which gives EV size distribution and concentration.[73,74] Nanoparticle tracking analysis can determine size distributions and concentrations, ranging in size from 50 nm to 1 micron.[75] Nanoparticle tracking analysis is slow and laborious, taking 10 minutes to measure 1000 particles. Additionally, optimization of camera and analysis settings is needed and vary depending on size of EVs measured.[24] Newer nanoparticle tracking analysis instruments can measure fluorescently labeled particles for biochemical analysis but it is not routinely used.[76] Finally, care should be taken during analysis phase of nanoparticle tracking analysis because it cannot distinguish between EVs and contaminants like lipoproteins or protein aggregates.[2]

Resistive pulse sensing
Resistive pulse sensing is commercially available as qNano (Izon Sciences). It gathers the size distribution and concentration by using the Coulter principle, which measures a change in ionic current as EVs are passed through a nanopore embedded in a membrane.[77,78] Resistive pulse sensing is also slow and laborious, taking 30 minutes to measure 1000 particles.[24] Additionally, to measure different size ranges of EVs, different nanopore filters have to be used.[2]

Dynamic light scattering
Dynamic light scattering, also known as photon correlation spectroscopy, calculates average size by measuring light scatter. Dynamic light scattering is not labor intensive and can measure EV concentrations quickly. Although dynamic light scattering can measure EV size ranging from 1 to 6 nm,[79] it is not recommended for determining distribution unless the EVs are monodisperse in size.[75]

Focus on Biochemical Analysis

Flow cytometry
Flow cytometry guides EVs in a hydrodynamic focused fluid stream pass a laser beam for detection.[75] Flow cytometry is a very powerful and quick method for determining EV concentration and biochemical properties; however, standardization has remained difficult. The original flow cytometry hurdle for EV characterization was the instruments' limited resolution (500 nm), because they were designed to analyze cells.[2] Therefore, EVs were coupled via antigen–antibody interactions to larger particles to analyze the presence of surface proteins. Newer flow cytometers have better resolution (100–200 nm), allowing larger individual EVs to be detected.[80–82] Additionally, finding appropriate sized standards with refractive indexes similar to EVs has been difficult.[83,84] This is critical to being able to reproduce measurements within a single and other laboratories. Finally, the analysis steps, such as gating, can vary significantly making standards even harder.[24]

Enzyme-linked immunosorbent assays
Enzyme-linked immunosorbent assays use antibodies that bind to EV surface antigens for capture, with detection occurring through another antibody–antigen interaction.[85] Although not used widely, kits for EV detection are sold by System Biosciences and Hansa BioMed. Functional assays are also available and more widely used.[48,66]

Western blots
Western blots are conventionally used to detect EVs by measuring EV-associated proteins.[86] A disadvantage of Western blots and enzyme-linked immunosorbent assays is that no individual EV measurement is done; rather, these techniques are limited to bulk

analysis. Finally, only the presence or enrichment of EV-associated proteins does not exclude that contaminants are absence.

Mass spectrometry

Mass spectrometry is another biochemical analysis method for EV detection and characterization and is being widely used for biomarker discovery. Mass spectrometry can detect EV-associated proteins, lipids, and metabolites by measuring the ion's mass to charge ratio. Mass spectrometry benefits from increased sensitivity and ability to analyze multiple proteins simultaneously.[87,88]

Biochemical analysis has focused on protein detection, with a subset of proteins used for EV detection. **Fig. 1** provides a list of identifying protein EV markers as they correlate to different EV species. Unfortunately, there is no clear consensus on specific nucleic acid EV identification markers. To detect EV nucleic acid cargo, traditional PCR, digital droplet PCR, microarrays, and next-generation sequencing have been explored.[1,61,89,90] The benefit of analyzing nucleic acids over proteins is that there is less background contaminating nucleic acid not associated with EVs as compared with proteins. It should also be noted that traditional PCR is another bulk measurement with the other nucleic acid detection methods able to measure individual molecules. There are now a few databases compiling protein, RNA, and lipid EV information from several studies into open source databases looking to identify functional markers, including Vesiclepedia,[91] EVpedia,[92] and ExoCarta.[93]

EXTRACELLULAR VESICLE CLINICAL SIGNIFICANCE

Although the exact physiologic functions of EVs are still poorly understood, they are widely known to act as transport vesicles for intercellular communication to maintain bodily homeostasis.[91] For example, EVs encapsulate messenger RNA and microRNA, with associated messenger RNA translated into protein when taken up by a target cell.[94,95] This EV cargo has also been found to be similar to the cells from which they originate. Consequently, these and similar findings have led EVs to be aggressively explored for diagnostic and therapeutic[96] applications, the latter of which are not discussed herein. Here, we briefly explore the diagnostic potential of EVs in oncology applications and discuss how Exosome Diagnostics is bringing them to the commercial market as laboratory developed tests (LDTs). It should be noted EVs are considered a liquid biopsy in addition to circulating tumor cells and cell-free nucleic acids, because they are all easily accessible from biofluids.

Tumor cells secrete EVs at a higher rate than that of normal cells and there is evidence they contribute to tumor progression, that is, invasion, intravasation, circulation, extravasation, and proliferation.[97,98] Tumor progression occurs through several mechanisms,[99,100] such as metastasis, microenvironment modifications,[101] immunosuppression, and promotion of angiogenesis. Tumor-associated EVs have also been shown to have antitumorigenic properties, like inducing tumor cell apoptosis.[102,103] Finally, tumor-associated EVs have also been found to have tumor-specific transcriptomic, genomic, and proteomic profiles.[98] **Table 1** shows a representation of promising cancer biomarkers isolated from EVs. More clinical studies with increased sample size are needed to further prove clinical usefulness.

At the time of this writing, 1 company has commercialized an EV-based LDT. The method uses an affinity column-based method to isolate EVs and their RNA contents.[61] This technology is sold as a kit through a partnership with Qiagen under the brand name exoEasy. Additionally, the company has developed another affinity column-based (exo52) EV isolation method that simultaneously captures cell free DNA and EV RNA but is not currently sold in a kit. The first EV-based diagnostic assay, ExoDx Lung

Table 1
Cancer biomarkers associated with extracellular vesicles

Cancer Type	Biomarker: Source Material	Clinical Biomarker Usefulness	Reference
Breast cancer	HER-2: protein	Monitoring	104
Glioblastoma	EGFR: protein, RNA	Diagnosis, prognosis monitoring	105,106
	Mutant IDH1: RNA	Diagnosis	64
Lung cancer	EGFR: protein	Prognosis	107,108
Melanoma	BRAFv700: RNA, DNA	Monitoring	109
Pancreatic cancer	KRAS, p53: DNA	Diagnosis, prognosis, monitoring	110
Prostate cancer	PSA, ERG: RNA	Diagnosis, monitoring	111,112

Abbreviations: EGFR, epidermal growth factor; PSA, prostate-specific antigen.
   Data from Refs.[64,104–112]

(ALK), was released in January 2016. It detects EML4-ALK variants, which is intended as a predictive driver of mutations in non–small cell lung cancer, from EV extracted RNA using reverse transcription quantitative PCR.[113–115] Exosome Diagnostics has also announced it will release 3 more EV-based diagnostics in 2016. Two assays will detect mutations in lung cancer, including, T790M resistance mutation (ExoDx Lung [T790M]) and epidermal growth factor activing mutations (ExoDx [epidermal growth factor]).[116–118] Both of these LDTs will also use circulating cell-free DNA and are detecting the mutations through targeted NGS to increase sensitivity. The final diagnostic assay (ExoDx Prostate [IntelliScore]) claims to provide key information on the aggressiveness of prostate cancer to avoid unnecessary solid tumor biopsies from a urine sample.[119–124] Aggressiveness is determined through a proprietary multivariate algorithm that integrates gene expression analysis of ERG and PCA3 normalized to SPDEF to produce a risk score. The current assays are offered as LDTs in their CLIA-certified laboratory, but they anticipate launching in vitro diagnostic test kits in the future following regulatory review. Although Exosome Diagnostics has focused on lung and prostate cancers, they have continued to publish abstracts describing other EV-based diagnostic assays for melanoma and colorectal cancer.[101,109,125]

SUMMARY

The interest in EVs has expanded rapidly as EVs were discovered to be abundantly present in different biofluids, contain nucleic acids, and participate in multiple regulatory functions.[1] This knowledge has posed EVs to have a significant role in the personalized medicine revolution, especially within the oncology field. The main advantages of EVs use in LDTs include:

- EVs are found in a variety of easily accessible biofluids, which allows frequent sampling;
- EVs have a molecular profile similar to their cellular origin;
- EV cargo is protected from degradation by a phospholipid membrane;
- EV fraction can remove other inhibitors found in biofluids that confound downstream analysis; and
- EVs better represent the heterogeneous nature of cancer because they collect in biofluids from multiple sites within and between tumors.

Overall, the information contained in EVs will potentially allow us to examine multiple clinical questions that are difficult to answer now, such as, who respond to a therapy, when resistance might develop, is there disease reoccurrence, and so on. Although what we know about EVs is increasing rapidly, much still needs to be done for EVs to reach their full potential as a source material in LDTs. We have touched on these challenges throughout and are summarized:

- Standardize EV nomenclature.
- Improve EV isolation purity and ability to separate different types of EVs.
- Develop an integrated method capable of EV detection and characterization.
- Further elucidate the physiologic role of EVs, that is, the biological mechanisms of packaging diagnostically relevant biomarkers.
- Is specificity and sensitivity acceptable for current downstream detection analytics?
- Can EVs be used in conjugation with circulating tumor cells or cell-free nucleic acids to further increase specificity and sensitivity of detecting diagnostically relevant biomarkers?

Many technical challenges remain and as such we are just beginning to scratch the clinical promise of EVs.

REFERENCES

1. Raposo G, Stoorvogel W. Extracellular vesicles: exosomes, microvesicles, and friends. J Cell Biol 2013;200(4):373–83.
2. Witwer KW, Buzás EI, Bemis LT, et al. Standardization of sample collection, isolation and analysis methods in extracellular vesicle research. J Extracell Vesicles 2013;2.
3. Chargaff E, West R. The biological significance of the thromboplastic protein of blood. J Biol Chem 1946;166(1):189–97.
4. Wolf P. The nature and significance of platelet products in human plasma. Br J Haematol 1967;13(3):269–88.
5. Dalton AJ. Microvesicles and vesicles of multivesicular bodies versus "virus-like" particles. J Natl Cancer Inst 1975;54(5):1137–48.
6. Johnstone RM, Adam M, Hammond JR, et al. Vesicle formation during reticulocyte maturation. Association of plasma membrane activities with released vesicles (exosomes). J Biol Chem 1987;262(19):9412–20.
7. Thery C, Zitvogel L, Amigorena S. Exosomes: composition, biogenesis and function. Nat Rev Immunol 2002;2(8):569–79.
8. Yanez-Mo M, Siljander PR, Andreu Z, et al. Biological properties of extracellular vesicles and their physiological functions. J Extracell Vesicles 2015;4: 27066.
9. Vlassov AV, Magdaleno S, Setterquist R, et al. Exosomes: current knowledge of their composition, biological functions, and diagnostic and therapeutic potentials. Biochim Biophys Acta 2012;1820(7):940–8.
10. Robbins PD, Morelli AE. Regulation of immune responses by extracellular vesicles. Nat Rev Immunol 2014;14(3):195–208.
11. Gould SJ, Raposo G. As we wait: coping with an imperfect nomenclature for extracellular vesicles. J Extracell Vesicles 2013;2.
12. Pan BT, Teng K, Wu C, et al. Electron microscopic evidence for externalization of the transferrin receptor in vesicular form in sheep reticulocytes. J Cell Biol 1985; 101(3):942–8.
13. Baietti MF, Zhang Z, Mortier E, et al. Syndecan-syntenin-ALIX regulates the biogenesis of exosomes. Nat Cell Biol 2012;14(7):677–85.

14. Colombo M, Moita C, van Niel G, et al. Analysis of ESCRT functions in exosome biogenesis, composition and secretion highlights the heterogeneity of extracellular vesicles. J Cell Sci 2013;126(Pt 24):5553–65.

15. Mathivanan S, Ji H, Simpson RJ. Exosomes: extracellular organelles important in intercellular communication. J Proteomics 2010;73(10):1907–20.

16. Muralidharan-Chari V, Clancy J, Plou C, et al. ARF6-regulated shedding of tumor cell-derived plasma membrane microvesicles. Curr Biol 2009;19(22):1875–85.

17. Li B, Antonyak MA, Zhang J, et al. RhoA triggers a specific signaling pathway that generates transforming microvesicles in cancer cells. Oncogene 2012; 31(45):4740–9.

18. Turiak L, Misják P, Szabó TG, et al. Proteomic characterization of thymocyte-derived microvesicles and apoptotic bodies in BALB/c mice. J Proteomics 2011;74(10):2025–33.

19. Di Vizio D, Morello M, Dudley AC, et al. Large oncosomes in human prostate cancer tissues and in the circulation of mice with metastatic disease. Am J Pathol 2012;181(5):1573–84.

20. Minciacchi VR, You S, Spinelli C, et al. Large oncosomes contain distinct protein cargo and represent a separate functional class of tumor-derived extracellular vesicles. Oncotarget 2015;6(13):11327–41.

21. Yuana Y, Böing AN, Grootemaat AE, et al. Handling and storage of human body fluids for analysis of extracellular vesicles. J Extracell Vesicles 2015;4:29260.

22. Lacroix R, Judicone C, Mooberry M, et al. Standardization of pre-analytical variables in plasma microparticle determination: results of the International Society on Thrombosis and Haemostasis SSC Collaborative workshop. J Thromb Haemost 2013;11(6):1190–3.

23. Lacroix R, Judicone C, Poncelet P, et al. Impact of pre-analytical parameters on the measurement of circulating microparticles: towards standardization of protocol. J Thromb Haemost 2012;10(3):437–46.

24. van der Pol E, Böing AN, Gool EL, et al. Recent developments in the nomenclature, presence, isolation, detection and clinical impact of extracellular vesicles. J Thromb Haemost 2016;14(1):48–56.

25. Lannigan J, P Nolan J, Zucker R. Measurement of extracellular vesicles and other submicron size particles by flow cytometry. Cytometry A 2016;89(2): 109–10.

26. Breddin HK, Harder S. The value of platelet function tests. Vasa 2003;32(3): 123–9.

27. Lippi G, Fontana R, Avanzini P, et al. Influence of mechanical trauma of blood and hemolysis on PFA-100 testing. Blood Coagul Fibrinolysis 2012;23(1):82–6.

28. Milburn JA, Ford I, Cassar K, et al. Platelet activation, coagulation activation and C-reactive protein in simultaneous samples from the vascular access and peripheral veins of haemodialysis patients. Int J Lab Hematol 2012;34(1):52–8.

29. Ayers L, Kohler M, Harrison P, et al. Measurement of circulating cell-derived microparticles by flow cytometry: sources of variability within the assay. Thromb Res 2011;127(4):370–7.

30. Satsangi J, Jewell DP, Welsh K, et al. Effect of heparin on polymerase chain reaction. Lancet 1994;343(8911):1509–10.

31. Maguire CA, Balaj L, Sivaraman S, et al. Microvesicle-associated AAV vector as a novel gene delivery system. Mol Ther 2012;20(5):960–71.

32. Gao C, Boylan B, Fang J, et al. Heparin promotes platelet responsiveness by potentiating alphaIIbbeta3-mediated outside-in signaling. Blood 2011;117(18): 4946–52.

33. Shah MD, Bergeron AL, Dong JF, et al. Flow cytometric measurement of microparticles: pitfalls and protocol modifications. Platelets 2008;19(5):365–72.
34. Gemmell CH, Sefton MV, Yeo EL. Platelet-derived microparticle formation involves glycoprotein IIb-IIIa. Inhibition by RGDS and a Glanzmann's thrombasthenia defect. J Biol Chem 1993;268(20):14586–9.
35. Momen-Heravi F, Balaj L, Alian S, et al. Impact of biofluid viscosity on size and sedimentation efficiency of the isolated microvesicles. Front Physiol 2012;3:162.
36. van Ierssel SH, Van Craenenbroeck EM, Conraads VM, et al. Flow cytometric detection of endothelial microparticles (EMP): effects of centrifugation and storage alter with the phenotype studied. Thromb Res 2010;125(4):332–9.
37. Trummer A, De Rop C, Tiede A, et al. Recovery and composition of microparticles after snap-freezing depends on thawing temperature. Blood Coagul Fibrinolysis 2009;20(1):52–6.
38. Dey-Hazra E, Hertel B, Kirsch T, et al. Detection of circulating microparticles by flow cytometry: influence of centrifugation, filtration of buffer, and freezing. Vasc Health Risk Manag 2010;6:1125–33.
39. Thery C, Amigorena S, Raposo G, et al. Isolation and characterization of exosomes from cell culture supernatants and biological fluids. Curr Protoc Cell Biol 2006;3:3.22.
40. Webber J, Clayton A. How pure are your vesicles? J Extracell Vesicles 2013;2.
41. Taylor DD, Shah S. Methods of isolating extracellular vesicles impact downstream analyses of their cargoes. Methods 2015;87:3–10.
42. Yuana Y, Levels J, Grootemaat A, et al. Co-isolation of extracellular vesicles and high-density lipoproteins using density gradient ultracentrifugation. J Extracell Vesicles 2014;3.
43. Muller L, Hong CS, Stolz DB, et al. Isolation of biologically-active exosomes from human plasma. J Immunol Methods 2014;411:55–65.
44. Cvjetkovic A, Lotvall J, Lasser C. The influence of rotor type and centrifugation time on the yield and purity of extracellular vesicles. J Extracell Vesicles 2014;3.
45. Zhang Z, Wang C, Li T, et al. Comparison of ultracentrifugation and density gradient separation methods for isolating Tca8113 human tongue cancer cell line-derived exosomes. Oncol Lett 2014;8(4):1701–6.
46. Palma J, Yaddanapudi SC, Pigati L, et al. MicroRNAs are exported from malignant cells in customized particles. Nucleic Acids Res 2012;40(18):9125–38.
47. Aalberts M, van Dissel-Emiliani FM, van Adrichem NP, et al. Identification of distinct populations of prostasomes that differentially express prostate stem cell antigen, annexin A1, and GLIPR2 in humans. Biol Reprod 2012;86(3):82.
48. Schageman J, Zeringer E, Li M, et al. The complete exosome workflow solution: from isolation to characterization of RNA cargo. Biomed Res Int 2013;2013: 253957.
49. Peterson MF, Otoc N, Sethi JK, et al. Integrated systems for exosome investigation. Methods 2015;87:31–45.
50. Taylor DD, Zacharias W, Gercel-Taylor C. Exosome isolation for proteomic analyses and RNA profiling. Methods Mol Biol 2011;728:235–46.
51. Yamada T, Inoshima Y, Matsuda T, et al. Comparison of methods for isolating exosomes from bovine milk. J Vet Med Sci 2012;74(11):1523–5.
52. Pisitkun T, Shen RF, Knepper MA. Identification and proteomic profiling of exosomes in human urine. Proc Natl Acad Sci U S A 2004;101(36):13368–73.
53. Gyorgy B, Módos K, Pállinger E, et al. Detection and isolation of cell-derived microparticles are compromised by protein complexes resulting from shared biophysical parameters. Blood 2011;117(4):e39–48.

54. Welton JL, Webber JP, Botos LA, et al. Ready-made chromatography columns for extracellular vesicle isolation from plasma. J Extracell Vesicles 2015;4:27269.

55. Boing AN, van der Pol E, Grootemaat AE, et al. Single-step isolation of extracellular vesicles by size-exclusion chromatography. J Extracell Vesicles 2014;3.

56. Kim G, Yoo CE, Kim M, et al. Noble polymeric surface conjugated with zwitterionic moieties and antibodies for the isolation of exosomes from human serum. Bioconjug Chem 2012;23(10):2114–20.

57. Yoo CE, Kim G, Kim M, et al. A direct extraction method for microRNAs from exosomes captured by immunoaffinity beads. Anal Biochem 2012;431(2):96–8.

58. Clayton A, Court J, Navabi H, et al. Analysis of antigen presenting cell derived exosomes, based on immuno-magnetic isolation and flow cytometry. J Immunol Methods 2001;247(1–2):163–74.

59. Tauro BJ, Greening DW, Mathias RA, et al. Comparison of ultracentrifugation, density gradient separation, and immunoaffinity capture methods for isolating human colon cancer cell line LIM1863-derived exosomes. Methods 2012; 56(2):293–304.

60. Cantin R, Diou J, Bélanger D, et al. Discrimination between exosomes and HIV-1: purification of both vesicles from cell-free supernatants. J Immunol Methods 2008;338(1–2):21–30.

61. Enderle D, Spiel A, Coticchia CM, et al. Characterization of RNA from exosomes and other extracellular vesicles isolated by a novel spin column-based method. PLoS One 2015;10(8):e0136133.

62. Liga A, Vliegenthart AD, Oosthuyzen W, et al. Exosome isolation: a microfluidic road-map. Lab Chip 2015;15(11):2388–94.

63. Shin H, Han C, Labuz JM, et al. High-yield isolation of extracellular vesicles using aqueous two-phase system. Sci Rep 2015;5:13103.

64. Chen C, Skog J, Hsu CH, et al. Microfluidic isolation and transcriptome analysis of serum microvesicles. Lab Chip 2010;10(4):505–11.

65. Lotvall J, Hill AF, Hochberg F, et al. Minimal experimental requirements for definition of extracellular vesicles and their functions: a position statement from the International Society for Extracellular Vesicles. J Extracell Vesicles 2014;3: 26913.

66. Erdbrugger U, Lannigan J. Analytical challenges of extracellular vesicle detection: a comparison of different techniques. Cytometry A 2016;89(2):123–34.

67. Raposo G, Nijman HW, Stoorvogel W, et al. B lymphocytes secrete antigen-presenting vesicles. J Exp Med 1996;183(3):1161–72.

68. Conde-Vancells J, Rodriguez-Suarez E, Embade N, et al. Characterization and comprehensive proteome profiling of exosomes secreted by hepatocytes. J Proteome Res 2008;7(12):5157–66.

69. Yuana Y, Koning RI, Kuil ME, et al. Cryo-electron microscopy of extracellular vesicles in fresh plasma. J Extracell Vesicles 2013;2.

70. Yuana Y, Oosterkamp TH, Bahatyrova S, et al. Atomic force microscopy: a novel approach to the detection of nanosized blood microparticles. J Thromb Haemost 2010;8(2):315–23.

71. Siedlecki CA, Wang IW, Higashi JM, et al. Platelet-derived microparticles on synthetic surfaces observed by atomic force microscopy and fluorescence microscopy. Biomaterials 1999;20(16):1521–9.

72. Ashcroft BA, de Sonneville J, Yuana Y, et al. Determination of the size distribution of blood microparticles directly in plasma using atomic force microscopy and microfluidics. Biomed Microdevices 2012;14(4):641–9.

73. Gardiner C, Ferreira YJ, Dragovic RA, et al. Extracellular vesicle sizing and enumeration by nanoparticle tracking analysis. J Extracell Vesicles 2013;2.
74. Filipe V, Hawe A, Jiskoot W. Critical evaluation of Nanoparticle Tracking Analysis (NTA) by NanoSight for the measurement of nanoparticles and protein aggregates. Pharm Res 2010;27(5):796–810.
75. van der Pol E, Hoekstra AG, Sturk A, et al. Optical and non-optical methods for detection and characterization of microparticles and exosomes. J Thromb Haemost 2010;8(12):2596–607.
76. Dragovic RA, Gardiner C, Brooks AS, et al. Sizing and phenotyping of cellular vesicles using Nanoparticle Tracking Analysis. Nanomedicine 2011;7(6):780–8.
77. Garza-Licudine E, Deo D, Yu S, et al. Portable nanoparticle quantization using a resizable nanopore instrument - the IZON qNano. Conf Proc IEEE Eng Med Biol Soc 2010;2010:5736–9.
78. de Vrij J, Maas SL, van Nispen M, et al. Quantification of nanosized extracellular membrane vesicles with scanning ion occlusion sensing. Nanomedicine (Lond) 2013;8(9):1443–58.
79. Dieckmann Y, Cölfen H, Hofmann H, et al. Particle size distribution measurements of manganese-doped ZnS nanoparticles. Anal Chem 2009;81(10):3889–95.
80. Lacroix R, Robert S, Poncelet P, et al. Overcoming limitations of microparticle measurement by flow cytometry. Semin Thromb Hemost 2010;36(8):807–18.
81. Robert S, Lacroix R, Poncelet P, et al. High-sensitivity flow cytometry provides access to standardized measurement of small-size microparticles–brief report. Arterioscler Thromb Vasc Biol 2012;32(4):1054–8.
82. van der Vlist EJ, Nolte-'t Hoen EN, Stoorvogel W, et al. Fluorescent labeling of nano-sized vesicles released by cells and subsequent quantitative and qualitative analysis by high-resolution flow cytometry. Nat Protoc 2012;7(7):1311–26.
83. Mullier F, Bailly N, Chatelain C, et al. More on: calibration for the measurement of microparticles: needs, interests, and limitations of calibrated polystyrene beads for flow cytometry-based quantification of biological microparticles. J Thromb Haemost 2011;9(8):1679–81 [author reply: 1681–2].
84. Chandler WL, Yeung W, Tait JF. A new microparticle size calibration standard for use in measuring smaller microparticles using a new flow cytometer. J Thromb Haemost 2011;9(6):1216–24.
85. Osumi K, Ozeki Y, Saito S, et al. Development and assessment of enzyme immunoassay for platelet-derived microparticles. Thromb Haemost 2001;85(2):326–30.
86. Abid Hussein MN, Nieuwland R, Hau CM, et al. Cell-derived microparticles contain caspase 3 in vitro and in vivo. J Thromb Haemost 2005;3(5):888–96.
87. Kreimer S, Belov AM, Ghiran I, et al. Mass-spectrometry-based molecular characterization of extracellular vesicles: lipidomics and proteomics. J Proteome Res 2015;14(6):2367–84.
88. Pocsfalvi G, Stanly C, Vilasi A, et al. Mass spectrometry of extracellular vesicles. Mass Spectrom Rev 2016;35(1):3–21.
89. Van Deun J, Mestdagh P, Sormunen R, et al. The impact of disparate isolation methods for extracellular vesicles on downstream RNA profiling. J Extracell Vesicles 2014;3.
90. Hill AF, Pegtel DM, Lambertz U, et al. ISEV position paper: extracellular vesicle RNA analysis and bioinformatics. J Extracell Vesicles 2013;2.

91. Kalra H, Kalra H, Simpson RJ, et al. Vesiclepedia: a compendium for extracellular vesicles with continuous community annotation. PLoS Biol 2012;10(12): e1001450.

92. Kim DK, Kang B, Kim OY, et al. EVpedia: an integrated database of high-throughput data for systemic analyses of extracellular vesicles. J Extracell Vesicles 2013;2.

93. Mathivanan S, Simpson RJ. ExoCarta: a compendium of exosomal proteins and RNA. Proteomics 2009;9(21):4997–5000.

94. Ratajczak J, Wysoczynski M, Hayek F, et al. Membrane-derived microvesicles: important and underappreciated mediators of cell-to-cell communication. Leukemia 2006;20(9):1487–95.

95. Valadi H, Ekström K, Bossios A, et al. Exosome-mediated transfer of mRNAs and microRNAs is a novel mechanism of genetic exchange between cells. Nat Cell Biol 2007;9(6):654–9.

96. Ohno S, Drummen GP, Kuroda M. Focus on extracellular vesicles: development of extracellular vesicle-based therapeutic systems. Int J Mol Sci 2016;17(2) [pii:E172].

97. Logozzi M, De Milito A, Lugini L, et al. High levels of exosomes expressing CD63 and caveolin-1 in plasma of melanoma patients. PLoS One 2009;4(4):e5219.

98. An T, Qin S, Xu Y, et al. Exosomes serve as tumour markers for personalized diagnostics owing to their important role in cancer metastasis. J Extracell Vesicles 2015;4:27522.

99. Rak J. Microparticles in cancer. Semin Thromb Hemost 2010;36(8):888–906.

100. Hood JL, San RS, Wickline SA. Exosomes released by melanoma cells prepare sentinel lymph nodes for tumor metastasis. Cancer Res 2011;71(11):3792–801.

101. Peinado H, Alečković M, Lavotshkin S, et al. Melanoma exosomes educate bone marrow progenitor cells toward a pro-metastatic phenotype through MET. Nat Med 2012;18(6):883–91.

102. Ristorcelli E, Beraud E, Verrando P, et al. Human tumor nanoparticles induce apoptosis of pancreatic cancer cells. FASEB J 2008;22(9):3358–69.

103. Zhang Y, Luo CL, He BC, et al. Exosomes derived from IL-12-anchored renal cancer cells increase induction of specific antitumor response in vitro: a novel vaccine for renal cell carcinoma. Int J Oncol 2010;36(1):133–40.

104. Ciravolo V, Huber V, Ghedini GC, et al. Potential role of HER2-overexpressing exosomes in countering trastuzumab-based therapy. J Cell Physiol 2012; 227(2):658–67.

105. Shao H, Chung J, Balaj L, et al. Protein typing of circulating microvesicles allows real-time monitoring of glioblastoma therapy. Nat Med 2012;18(12):1835–40.

106. Skog J, Würdinger T, van Rijn S, et al. Glioblastoma microvesicles transport RNA and proteins that promote tumour growth and provide diagnostic biomarkers. Nat Cell Biol 2008;10(12):1470–6.

107. Park JO, Choi DY, Choi DS, et al. Identification and characterization of proteins isolated from microvesicles derived from human lung cancer pleural effusions. Proteomics 2013;13(14):2125–34.

108. Yamashita T, Kamada H, Kanasaki S, et al. Epidermal growth factor receptor localized to exosome membranes as a possible biomarker for lung cancer diagnosis. Pharmazie 2013;68(12):969–73.

109. Sullivan RJ, O'Neill VJ, Enderle D, et al. Plasma-based monitoring of braf mutations during therapy for malignant melanoma using combined exosomal RNA and cell-free DNA Analysis. In American Society of Clinical Oncology Annual Meeting. Chicago, IL, May 29-June 2, 2015.

110. Kahlert C, Melo SA, Protopopov A, et al. Identification of double-stranded genomic DNA spanning all chromosomes with mutated KRAS and p53 DNA in the serum exosomes of patients with pancreatic cancer. J Biol Chem 2014; 289(7):3869–75.

111. Donovan MJ, Noerholm M, Bentink S, et al. A molecular signature of PCA3 and ERG exosomal RNA from non-DRE urine is predictive of initial prostate biopsy result. Prostate Cancer Prostatic Dis 2015;18(4):370–5.

112. Nilsson J, Skog J, Nordstrand A, et al. Prostate cancer-derived urine exosomes: a novel approach to biomarkers for prostate cancer. Br J Cancer 2009;100(10): 1603–7.

113. Brinkmann K, Emenegger J, Carbone D, et al. Exosomal RNA-based liquid biopsy detection of EML4-ALK in plasma from NSCLC patients. In National Comprehensive Cancer Network 21st Annual Conference. Hollywood, FL, March 31, 2016.

114. Brinkmann K, Emenegger J, Carbone D, et al. Noerholm Exosomal RNA-based liquid biopsy detection of EML4-ALK in plasma from NSCLC patients. In 2015 IASLC 16th World Conference on Lung Cancer. Denver, CO, September 6-9, 2015.

115. Brinkmann K, Enderle D, Koestler T, et al. Plasma-based diagnostics for detection of EML4-ALK fusion transcripts in NSCLC patients. In 2015 American Association for Cancer Research Annual Meeting. Philadelphia, April 18-22, 2015.

116. Krug AK, Karlovich C, Koestler T, et al. Plasma EGFR mutation detection using a combined exosomal RNA and circulating tumor DNA approach in patients with acquired resistance to first-generation EGFR-TKIs. In 26th AACR-NCI-EORTC International Conference on Molecular Targets and Cancer Therapeutics. Boston, MA, November 5-9, 2015.

117. Krug AK, Koestler T, Enderle D, et al. EGFR activating and T790M resistance mutation in plasma exoRNA and cfDNA, detected with single-step isolation columns and targeted resequencing. In 2015 IASLC 16th World Conference on Lung Cancer. Denver, CO, September 6-9, 2015.

118. O'Neill VJ, Brinkmann K, Enderle D, et al. Detection of EGFR activating and T790M resistance mutation in plasma of NSCLC patients using combined exosomal RNA and cfDNA capture. Presented at the 16th Annual International Lung Cancer Congress. Huntington Beach, CA, July 30-August 1, 2015.

119. Donovan MJ, Noerholm M, Bentink S, et al. Interim performance of a non-DRE urine exosome gene signature to predict Gleason $\geq$7 prostate cancer on initial prostate needle biopsy from patients enrolled in a prospective observational trial. In 2015 American Society of Clinical Oncology Annual Meeting. Chicago, IL, May 29-June 2, 2015.

120. McKiernan J. Validation of a novel non-invasive urine exosome gene expression assay to predict high-grade prostate cancer in patients undergoing initial biopsy with an equivocal PSA. Presented at the 2015 American Urological Association Annual Meeting. New Orleans, LA, May 15-19, 2015.

121. Donovan MJ, Noerholm M, Bentink S, et al. A first catch, non-DRE urine exosome gene signature to predict Gleason 7 prostate cancer on an initial prostate needle biopsy. Presented at the 2015 Genitourinary Cancers Symposium. Orlando, FL, February 26-28, 2015.

122. Donovan M, Bentink S, Noerholm KM, et al. Extended analysis of a validated urine-exosome signature to predict high grade prostate cancer on initial biopsy maintains performance across multiple sub-groups. In Genitourinary Cancers Symposium. San Francisco, CA, January 7-9, 2016.

123. Donovan M, Eastham J, Patel V, et al. A non-invasive urine exosome gene expression assay (ExoIntelliScoreTM Prostate) accurately predicts pathological stage and grade in the prostatectomy specimen. In Genitourinary Cancers Symposium. San Francisco, CA, January 7-9, 2016.
124. Hurley J, Hu L, Brock G, et al. A non-invasive urine exosome gene expression assay (ExoIntelliScore Prostate) accurately predicts pathologic stage and grade in the prostatectomy specimen. In 18th European Cancer Congress. Vienna, Austria, September 25-29, 2015.
125. Enderle D, Koestler T, Sullivan RJ, et al. Monitoring therapy response and resistance mutations in circulating RNA and DNA of plasma from melanoma patients. In 26th EORTC-NCI-AACR Symposium on Molecular Targets and Cancer Therapeutic. Barcelona, Spain, November 18-21, 2014.

Moving?

Make sure your subscription moves with you!

To notify us of your new address, find your **Clinics Account Number** (located on your mailing label above your name), and contact customer service at:

Email: journalscustomerservice-usa@elsevier.com

800-654-2452 (subscribers in the U.S. & Canada)
314-447-8871 (subscribers outside of the U.S. & Canada)

Fax number: 314-447-8029

Elsevier Health Sciences Division
Subscription Customer Service
3251 Riverport Lane
Maryland Heights, MO 63043

*To ensure uninterrupted delivery of your subscription, please notify us at least 4 weeks in advance of move.

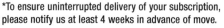

Printed and bound by CPI Group (UK) Ltd, Croydon, CR0 4YY

03/10/2024

01040397-0015